ONE HABIT AT A TIME

9 ESSENTIAL HABITS FOR A TALLER, BRIGHTER AND HAPPIER YOU

By: Salvatore Crispo

ONE HABIT AT A TIME

Copyright © 2010 by Salvatore Crispo

All rights reserved.

This book or any portion thereof may not be reproduced or used in any manner whatsoever without the express written permission of the publisher except for the use of brief quotations in a book review.

ISBN: 978-0-9866320-0-6
Crispo, Salvatore

www.habitwatch.ca

Table of Contents

ACKNOWLEDGEMENTS	i
NOTE FROM THE EDITOR	iv
FOREWORD	vii
PREFACE	xii
INTRODUCTION	1

PART 1: ESSENTIAL HABITS FOR THE PHYSICAL BODY

CH.1	POSTURE – The Habit Of Good Posture	9
CH.2	BREATHE – The Habit Of High-Quality Breathing	28
CH.3	SMILE – The Habit Of Smiling	50

PART 2: ESSENTIAL HABITS FOR THE MIND

CH.4	MINDFULNESS – The Habit of Being Mindful	71
CH.5	THINK – The Habit Of Accurate Thinking	94
CH.6	ACTION – The Habit Of Affirmative Action	118

ONE HABIT AT A TIME

PART 3: ESSENTIAL HABITS FOR THE SPIRIT

CH.7	CONNECTEDNESS – The Habit Of Conscious Unity	145
CH.8	GRATEFULNESS – The Habit Of Giving Thanks	175
CH.9	GOLDEN RULE – The Habit Of Service	193
	CONCLUSION	214

Acknowledgements

Family

Caterina Crispo: To an all-giving Mother, for your nurturing, your love and your faith. Thank you for always supporting me in everything I do.

Nicola Crispo: A great soul equals a great Father. You have taught me through example, more than anyone else in this world, how to express love. Thank you for this and your constant love.

Rosa Crispo: To my lovely sister who has taught me to have the courage to be my authentic-self.

Franca Infusino: To my wife, you are the love of my life! We are on an exhilarating journey together and I am grateful for every second that we share. I love you!

Julian Crispo: A special bond transpired between us at your birth that ensured me we would be connected forever. This book is dedicated to you and all the children of this world.

ONE HABIT AT A TIME

Editors

Luca Ciciarelli: To Luca for proof reading and editing this book. Your skills are unmatched when it comes to the way you conducted this special service. Often, it is not easy for a creator to listen to criticism of their creation, but you criticized with such gentleness and class that you transformed this daunting process into a joyful experience. Your generosity will never be forgotten. Working by your side is an honour and simply having you in my life is a great blessing. From the depths of my heart, thank you.

Salvatore Ciciarelli: To Sal for proof reading this book. Your feedback is always held in the highest regard. You have taught me to express myself carefully so that I would always leave the readers with a choice and not a command. Thank you for always being there when ever I need you.

Marco Racco: I consider you my spiritual brother. Thank you for always believing in me, encouraging me to shine, and bringing out the best in me. I look forward to living our dream of bringing holistic health to the world.

Design Specialist

Eric Favata: You are a true professional in every sense of the word. I always enjoy watching you work your magic on the computer. Your creations are sheer brilliance which is exemplified in the design the Habit Watch logo and website.

ACKNOWLEDGEMENTS

Mentors

Salvatore Crispo: To my late Grandfather, who showed me the value of character and set a great example for me to emulate. I will always love you.

Paul Chek: You are by far one of the most extraordinary people I know. No one has had more of an impact on my education than you. Your teachings have helped me (as well as thousands of others) to transform my life into what it is today and for this I am forever grateful. Also, thank you for taking the time out of your extremely busy schedule to write the foreword for this book.

Note from the Editor

"Such as are your habitual thoughts, such also will be the character of your mind; for the soul is dyed by the thoughts."

~ Marcus Aurelius Antoninus
(26 April 121 – 17 March 180, Roman Emperor)

     Such profound words dating back almost two thousand years. The struggle that humanity has with *habit* is impervious to the transcendence of time. Somewhat of a mystery, somewhat obvious…if we can form bad habits with relative ease, then why can't we form goods ones just as easily?
     We all know that life is always changing, and we are faced with new challenges almost on a daily basis. These challenges quite often lead to stress build up. In certain cases, the stress can become so extreme, that it interferes with our abilities to perform even routine daily activities. It is this very stress that can lead to the development of negative habits. So a big part of developing new, positive habits has a great deal to do with managing your stress levels. It is crucial to bring our stress

NOTE FROM THE EDITOR

levels under control, as many recent studies have shown that stress has contributed to high blood pressure, lack of concentration, digestive issues and longer recovery times from illness or injury, just to name a few. This then begs the question, "can stress be managed, and if so, how?"

Well, the following book written by Sal Crispo, delves into the process of habit formation. His easy to understand, step-by-step approach provides not only great advice on how to create new, positive habits, but explains how easy it can actually be to incorporate these approaches into your everyday life. All of the techniques laid out in this book, whether directly or indirectly, deal with managing your stress levels. Once you can take charge of your stress levels, you will find significant improvement in even the smallest aspects of your life whether at home, in your social life or your professional life.

With the assistance of *One Habit At A Time* and the Habit Watch, achieving your goals will be made easy. Whether these goals are physical, mental, emotional or spiritual, anyone can experience considerable development in all aspects of their life. And if you were to encounter any difficulties or road-blocks during your journey, you will not be left to fend for yourself, as the author has provided additional resources and contact information so that he can personally help to guide you in the right direction, putting you back on track towards achieving what you may have thought previously impossible.

As I read through this body of work, it quickly became apparent that the author also considers that we are all unique, we are individuals with individual needs, so the book is presented in a way that everyone can follow, so that they may proceed at their own pace. If you can create certain positive habits more quickly, then by all means, read on. If you require more time, then take it! And if there is a certain habit that you would like to revisit, simply go back and re-read that chapter…it's that simple. Also, the language used is one of straightforwardness and ease. Being written in such an uncomplicated and unambiguous manner is intentional, so that any reader can understand all of the author's ideas and intentions, allowing for everyone to benefit from this process.

In closing, I would just like to say that I have had the privilege of knowing Sal his entire life. I have come to trust him implicitly because of the determination that he demonstrates each and every day. He has an unsurpassed dedication to his field of study, has conducted countless hours of research and has been trained by none other than Paul Chek, one of the foremost health experts in the world. He is a caring husband, loving father, consummate professional and becomes a best friend to everyone who is fortunate enough to meet him. He never backs down from a challenge and chose this field of study because he truly wants to make a difference in people's lives by always being willing to lend a hand or offer great, sound advice. The list of those he has helped is long and growing with each passing day. I am glad that you now have decided to join this list by reading his work. I assure you that you have nothing to lose and everything to gain. Enjoy!

Luca Mario Ciciarelli
Entrepreneur
University of Toronto, *B.A.*

"We first make our habits, and then our habits make us."

~ John Dryden
(9 August 1631 – 12 May 1700, influential English poet)

Foreword

  If you are reading this, you are on a journey called "LIFE". Most of us spend the whole of our journey fearing death...does that ever really add any quality to your life experience, or just keep you looking for what you "don't want"? Sadly, most of us were raised in families whose ideology was steeped in religious traditionalism. That traditionalism, unfortunately, is a muddle of control, confusion, conflict and produces exactly what it is designed to produce by those detached from the wisdom, intention, passion and motives of the founding Fathers. When repentance must come by way of the saviour, church, the priest, the father (figure), and it is made profitable, the business of religion begins, and the practice of being spiritual is subverted.

  To the degree that we judge our natural desires for intimacy, self-exploration, creativity, abundance, or even dreaming as wrong, selfish, shameful, hedonistic, we are likely to instill guilt and shame programs within our psyche. Once we accept the ideas of any outsider, we become a reflection of our acceptance. What does that look like? You don't have to walk far to find a god-fearing Muslim, Christian, or one of Jewish faith that will agree with you that, God Is Love, or that God Is All. However, most people will deny that if God is God, then all that there can be in the Universe IS GOD! They need a "good god" to counterbalance (their) "devils".

ONE HABIT AT A TIME

The result of such cross-wiring is the creation of "gods", which leads to "my god vs. your god" consciousness; it leads to people worshiping God, yet, voting for leaders that condone war against the "infidels", or the "terrorists", or the "Jews", or the "Palestinians", or the "other." To the very degree that we participate in such systems of belief, we create angels and demons within ourselves. When we watch anyone being mistreated, by our impetus, or that of another, we feel the pain within. If we have not developed a healthy sense of self, which can't occur without an open mind, we go into denial as a means of self-protection.

Soon, your soul leads you to a book like *One Habit At A Time*. Then, you may experience an awakening. That awakening, to the degree that it is profound, comes with self-reflection. True self-reflection delineates self-responsibility. Many people will be afraid to make the kind of changes Sal Crispo offers here in *One Habit At A Time* for fear of becoming different than the family, tribe, pack, or society; what will they think of me if I stop going to church? What will they think of me if they find out I've been reading Buddhist books? Who will believe me when I tell them I've found "Christ Consciousness within myself"? If you are not ready to be an individual, an individual in the healthiest sense of the word, then you will find the attempts to heal to be an unbearable burden; that burden is one every ego must go through to get to the light shining within.

If fear guides your decisions, you will most likely go into inner-turmoil; you will know the truths of *One Habit At A Time* are real, yet, you will know that you are not living them (again!). The result is that you create and run a "denial" program in your head to justify your self-induced ignorance of the truth. The more you do this, the more conflicted you get and this conflict, to the degree that it is suppressed, acts like weeds in an untended garden -

FORWORD

soon they strangle the flowers and the fruits such that the potential harvest seems an unbearable task.

This suppression or denial manifests in our body as a blockage to the natural flow of life~force and leads first to pain, then to illness, then to disease, and often, to death. If along the way, your loved ones, friends, therapists or doctors identify where you are in denial (which usually occurs because addictive behaviours are railroading your hopes and dreams), you are likely to create denial of denial programs. This common progression leads to a very sad state of existence. It is as though your life is one long court trial and the headlines read, "The World Against Me!" This is the path to depression, chronic fatigue, and apathy. It need not be that way!

This beautiful book, *One Habit At A Time* offers you exactly that, the ability to create your "True Self" through conscious awareness. That effectively takes place one habit at a time! Whenever we become brave enough, honest enough to look into the mirror of "self," we first see what we think we are. Then, as we choose to live our dreams, we begin to see another person in the (same) mirror. They are taller, brighter, happier, more willing to rest and nurture themselves, for now, they have both hope and a reason to get out of bed. With a dream, we have a reason to participate in life and to share the love we create within ourselves, with others. After all, if we can't share our love, what's it really for?

Having love and passion and not being able to share it is but another form of solitary confinement. Love not shared begins to hurt. When we come to realize that indeed, we are sharing our love (how ever it may manifest) wherever we go, we eventually accept responsibility for the fact that all we can pass onto others is what we are, what we've become. Soon, we come to realize that all we can take with us when we leave this world is what we have become; cars, money, houses, etc., don't fit through the eye of that needle!

Because the truth of all life is that Unconditional Love (SOUL) is its source, substance and sustenance, we can choose to see that light within not only every "being", but every "thing", for if God is God, then God IS ALL there IS. It is my dream that everyone that reads this wonderful book, *One Habit At A Time*, chooses to let the light of Love and Life shine through them, like a light through a prism. When we choose to be present with the light, we can, out of self-honesty, see where the metaphorical windows need some cleaning. When we know Love is our essential nature, our True-Self, then we are not only willing to share our love, passions and dreams, we are willing to polish our windows so we can see that love both outside us, and make it easier for others to see and feel that love within us.

The journey to peace, bliss, and unadulterated consciousness that all world religions intended to share as an expression of the love and wisdom of their founders is a journey of converting one faulty belief and/or behaviour at a time. Just think how different your life would be if you just allowed yourself to experience the belief that God IS LOVE, and not something to fear. If the highest form of love is Unconditional, can there really be a judgment day? Can you really be a sinner? Can you really be a bad person? Or could these beliefs just be the rocks under which an invaluable treasure is buried so you and all in your life can rejoice and share when you find it?

I personally embrace Sal Crispo's beautiful book, *One Habit At A Time* because as the old saying goes, a journey of a thousand miles begins with the first step. Sal has shared the wisdom of many "great lights" and has done so not as a stenographer or a parrot, but out of his own authentic experience of changing one habit at a time. This book is Sal's love being offered to you. It is the very nature

FORWORD

of love to include. No matter how you cultivate love in your life, you will find it the most infectious of gifts. What you learn and experience in application of the methods in this book will shine from your very pores. You will not have to do anything to fix people. No, indeed, as you clean your own windows and begin seeing through the eyes of LOVE, you will indeed see that all that was once ugly to you, becomes beautiful. You will come to realize that because GOD can only be Unconditional LOVE (anything else suggests "needs", which contradicts SELF-SUFFICIENCY or GODLINESS), everyone is getting exactly what they wish (or pray) for with greatest frequency and intensity (thoughts!). You will see that nothing needs fixing. You will come to love and allow naturally, all without needing to kill or eradicate those with opposing viewpoints. You will, one habit at a time, find yourself looking right into a Divine Mirror. There, you will know that the best thing to do with a mirror reflecting such magnificent beauty (the Universe!) is polish it and share the light with all.

    I encourage each of you to live your dreams, for in so doing, the love will naturally rise, emerge and all the dark spots within transform in such light. Soon, you will come to realize that if God is God, then there can be no death, for God can't die and as Prime Source, all we can possibly be is God! Let's do "Godliness" together, One Habit At A Time!

Love and chi,

Paul Chek
Holistic Health Practitioner
Author, *How to Eat, Move and Be Healthy!*
Founder, The C.H.E.K. Institute
San Diego, CA

Preface

"The ideas I stand for are not mine. I borrowed them from Socrates. I swiped them from Chesterfield. I stole them from Jesus. And I put them in a book. If you don't like their rules, whose would you use?"

~ Dale Carnegie

Welcome fellow reader! You are about to embark on a special journey, a journey of self-discovery, self-growth and self-transformation. And the beauty of this journey is that it is on-going. For you can always learn more about yourself, you can always advance to higher levels in all facets of life, and finally, you can always reshape your habits, character, and destiny. What's more, you can begin doing any of these three things at any moment as it is never too late to start improving your life.

For as long as I can remember, I have had a strong inclination to help others improve their life and it is for this reason that I have written this book. In order to effectively help others, I have used the same approach in this book that I use as a holistic health practitioner. A holistic health practitioner uses a holistic approach to health and wellness. This approach has a profound and life-changing impact on people. This is because the holistic approach to health and wellness beautifully integrates the body, mind, and spirit.

PREFACE

A holistic health practitioner knows that the root cause of almost all stress, suffering and unhappiness, etc., is due to the neglect of one or more of these 3 main areas (body, mind, and spirit). Therefore, the holistic health practitioner's role is to teach others how to live a happy and healthy life by helping them to develop a balanced focus on the growth or development of all 3 of these areas.

As a holistic health practitioner, it has become my mission to teach as many people as possible how to live a holistically balanced lifestyle. In order to live such a balanced lifestyle, one must learn to adopt certain principles or habits. In this book, I present 9 (3 physical, 3 mental and 3 spiritual) of the most important habits one can adopt to live a happy and healthy life. What's more, I will teach you how to use a tried, tested and true method that will allow you to build these habits with relative ease. I am very excited about sharing this simple and practical method with you.

Simplicity and practicality carry a lot of value in our modern day society. We lead more complex lives (careers, education, families, etc.) than ever before. As a result, there are a lot more distractions today than at any other time in history. These distractions can pull us in all sorts of directions causing us to end up in unfavourable life situations. However, this easy-to-use method allows anyone to maintain control of their life in order to create the life of their dreams.

You may notice that I use a writing style that maintains the theme of simplicity and practicality. I chose this approach because I strongly believe in the saying that 'clarity leads to power'. I knew that in order for this book to have a powerful impact on the lives of the readers, it had to be clear. Therefore, I have taken a lot of valuable information and organized it in a unique fashion so that it may be clearly understood by everyone. Once understood,

ONE HABIT AT A TIME

this information can be easily implemented into your life with the method you will learn of in this book. I am aware that all information can be rebutted. Therefore, I have tried, for the most part, to present this information as common knowledge or common sense. I have gathered information that I firmly believe can be constructive to anyone who chooses to use it as directed. Furthermore, I have supported the information presented by using many quotes from some of the wisest men and women whose presence has graced this planet. And finally, if the reader is still not convinced that my recipe for self-discovery, self-growth and self-transformation will work to improve their life, I only ask that they give it a try.

You have nothing to lose and everything to gain! There is virtually little to no financial cost to using this method. You are using something that you already possess and it passes you by anyway - TIME. I welcome you to try and prove this method wrong because I am confident that it will sufficiently prove its own self-worth. In truth, if you want to improve your health, achieve financial freedom, create wonderful relationships, or realize whatever your heart desires then this book will show you how to do so.

Yours truly,

Sal Crispo

Introduction

THE HABIT WATCH

"*A consciousness of wrongdoing is the first step to salvation…you have to catch yourself doing it before you can correct it.*"

~ Seneca

Many of us know that good habits usually bring good results and poor habits usually bring poor results. But sometimes habits are hard to change. That is because most habits are being done **unconsciously**. Let me give you an example of exactly what I mean by 'being done unconsciously'. A few years ago I had the habit of biting my fingernails. I really hated this habit. I remember being so embarrassed of my fingernails that I would hide them from others at school, work and social gatherings. For many years, I tried to break the habit without any success.
      The main reason I had difficulty breaking this habit was because I would bite my fingernails without realizing I

ONE HABIT AT A TIME

was doing so. It is similar to the experience of catching yourself singing a song you do not like. You ask yourself, *'Why am I singing this song? How long have I been singing it for?'* Most likely, you do not know the answers to these questions because you are doing it unconsciously. It is in this state of unconsciousness that we are most inclined to do that which we habitually do. Conversely, when we are in a **conscious** state, then we have the ability to choose to continue or change what we are doing. A saying that I learned from Robin Sharma, author of *"The Monk Who Sold His Ferrari"*, is "awareness precedes choice which then precedes change."

Therefore, it is my belief that changing or creating a new habit would be more easily accomplished if we could stay conscious throughout the day. What does it mean to become or stay conscious? Simply put, it means to be alert, aware or fully present of the moment. In other words, it is a heightened sense of awareness, one that is very difficult for most people to remain in. However, with some daily practice, you can easily build this extremely important habit of heightened awareness.

In the eastern-world, they refer to this practice of awareness as **meditation**. Many of the eastern cultures practice meditation everyday because they know and understand its great importance. Most people visualize meditation as sitting on the floor in complete silence. This sitting meditation is a great way to begin practicing awareness. However, the real challenge of practicing awareness or staying conscious is when we are dealing with our real life situations.

Can we learn to stay in this state of consciousness…when we are at work? When we are with our friends on a night out? When we are in an argument with a loved one? I believe this to be the most difficult and advanced form of meditation to learn. But also the most important! For this reason, I have devised a simple and

INTRODUCTION

practical means for anyone to develop the habit of advanced awareness no matter what the circumstance.

As a holistic health practitioner and CHEK practitioner (CHEK institute), I use the following method to correct peoples' posture. I have my clients set their watches to beep once every 15, 30, or 60 minutes. This one beep reminds them to check their current posture and change it if they find themselves in a poor postural position. I refer to this timed method as '**The Habit Watch Method**'. Using the Habit Watch is amazing because it reminds them to re-adjust their posture (if necessary) throughout the day. This method effectively aids my clients in improving their posture.

How does the Habit Watch aid my clients exactly? Well, I understood that once a client left their 1 hour session of postural corrective training, they were going back to their real life situations. A common, real life example of this is sitting in front of a computer all day long and dealing with a stressful job. It is more likely that they are thinking about work and not their posture. I knew this was a problem because it would be extremely difficult to overcome 12 or more hours of poor postural habits with only 1 hour a day of postural correction. Therefore, the Habit Watch became a great tool for me in managing the habitual patterns of my clients even when I was not physically with them.

The results I attained from the Habit Watch were so profound for correcting postural habits that its use naturally progressed toward all sorts of other habits. In this book, I present to you 9 life changing habits. I chose these 9 habits because I believe them to be the most important habits for anyone to build. They will bring success to all areas of your life and they will help support you in building more constructive habits in the future. There is an endless amount of positive habits to develop in a lifetime and the

ONE HABIT AT A TIME

Habit Watch will prove to be a proficient tool for habit development.

I would like to stress the reason why the Habit Watch is so effective. Every time the watch beeps (or vibrates) it wakes you up if you have fallen into a state of mental unconsciousness. It is the same as an alarm clock. An alarm clock is designed to wake you up from sleep at a specific time. This ensures that you do not sleep in and miss out on whatever it is you have planned for that day. In a similar manner, the Habit Watch ensures that you do not forget about the new habit you are trying to create. It is a wake-up call into a higher state of consciousness or awareness. It allows you to step outside of yourself and – WATCH YOUR HABITS! (This is my cheeky slogan for the Habit Watch)

To further explain the meaning of a higher state of consciousness, I will use my former habit of fingernail biting as an example. I would often catch myself chewing on my fingernails while watching hockey on television. Although I was awake or conscious enough to be watching the game, I was not in a higher state of awareness to realize that I was also biting on my fingernails. As soon as I did **realize** (entered into a higher state of consciousness) what I was doing then I made a conscious choice to stop because I wanted to quit. It took me until the 25th year of my life to truly grasp what this higher state of consciousness (awareness, being, etc.) really meant. So do not worry if it is a little confusing. I will expand on this topic throughout the book, especially in chapter 4 – The habit of being mindful.

Here is a brief outline of the structure of this book. There are 3 main parts to the book – Physical, Mental, and Spiritual. Each part contains 3 habits (chapters) to be developed. Each chapter is divided into 3 main parts. After a short introduction, I give a description of WHAT the habit is exactly. Second, I explain WHY the habit is so

INTRODUCTION

important to develop and I list the benefits of doing so. And finally, I show you HOW to effectively develop the habit.

Here are some guidelines on how this book should be used. I recommend you read this book in its entirety without attempting to master the habits. This will allow you to better understand how each habit connects to the other. Once you have read the book in its entirety, you can go back and reread the chapter of the first habit to be mastered. After mastering a habit, you can move on to the next one.

Careful thought was used to establish the order of the habits I chose for this book. Therefore, I also recommend that the reader follows each habit in the order they are presented. For example, I chose to begin with the habit of good posture and not with the habit of high-quality breathing because a person can breathe more efficiently if first they are in a good postural position. All of the habits presented are linked and they flow in a logical manner. Each habit builds upon and supports the previous habit(s).

Take your time learning and developing each habit. Only move onto the next habit when you feel that you have a good sense of control of the current habit. You will know you have developed a habit when the Habit Watch beeps and you already find yourself practicing it most of the time (at least 80% of the time). After mastering each habit, it is not forgotten but it is added to your mental checklist. When the Habit Watch beeps, you will learn to check through all the habits you have developed to see if you are doing them at that moment.

You are now ready to begin your journey through this book. I will be with you in Spirit until the end. My heart and soul are on these pages. I have lain before you information that I believe, if followed, will lead you to a more healthy, loving, and successful life. Please, enjoy the

ONE HABIT AT A TIME

rest of the book and remember – change your habits and you will change your life!

Part I

THREE ESSENTIAL HABITS FOR THE PHYSICAL BODY

"The mind's first step to self-awareness must be through the body."

~ **George Sheehan**

1

Posture

THE HABIT OF GOOD POSTURE

"The omnipresence of habit is almost terrifying when one reflects upon it. From the minute a man shuts off his alarm clock on one morning, till the minute he shuts it off on the next morning, it controls him. It dictates and makes possible nine-tenths of his actions. And nine-tenths of the habits of most men are formed unconsciously.
It is astounding that men should so leave this thing to chance, when it determines the very texture of their lives; yet the fact must be recorded."

~ Henry Hazlitt

All habits are learned and exist because of a conscious or unconscious choice. I have realized that habits are created, for the most part, by unconscious choices. This is most apparent in the boy who emulates his

ONE HABIT AT A TIME

father. He imitates his father's posture, gait, mannerisms, etc., without realizing he does so. Although it is adorable to see the boy imitating his father, the problem lies in that not all learned habits are positive. The boy takes on his father's negative habits too and someday will pass them on to his children.

To prevent this generational cycle of negative habits, the boy must eventually become conscious of all his habits and decide whether or not he wishes to keep them. If the boy does not want to keep certain habits in his life, there are several ways he can get rid of them. I believe that the most effective method to rid a negative habit is to consciously replace it with its opposite. For example; in this opening chapter you will be learning about developing the opposite habit of poor posture – good posture. And remember, when you replace a negative habit with its positive counterpart, your life will change for the better.

There are various reasons why the habit of good posture is the foundation of the 9 habits presented in this book. There is an old saying, 'how we do one thing is how we do everything'. In other words, how well you master the habit of good posture usually indicates how well you will build other habits. With that being said, I am not asking you to do the impossible. All you must do is put a reasonable amount of effort into developing each habit and you will see incredible results and transformations. In addition, one of the most difficult tasks for developing a habit will be done for you by the Habit Watch – periodically reminding you to practice the habit that you are developing.

It is more difficult to see progression, change or results in certain habits. For the most part, it is far easier to see physical transformations than mental or spiritual ones. For instance, it is very simple to determine whether or not you are in good posture. You are either upright or you are not. For this reason, I chose to present and build the physical habits first. Why is it important that you are able to see results? Well, when you begin to catch yourself in a good postural position more often, you will start to understand the power of the Habit Watch Method. Thus, as you begin to experience results with building the habit of good posture, it will motivate you to build many more habits using this method.

WHAT IS THE HABIT OF GOOD POSTURE?

Good Posture & Poor Posture

In this chapter, I use the terms 'good posture' when describing a person being in an upright position and 'poor posture' when describing a person being in a slouched position. I am aware that there is much more to good posture than simply keeping upright, however, there can be a significant difference made in a person's life by simply creating the habit of being upright versus being slouched. The section at the end of this chapter, 'going the extra mile with the habit of good posture', is for any reader who wishes to delve deeper into the extensive subject of creating good posture. However, it is highly recommended that all readers should explore and learn more about posture. Here are two images, followed by a technical description of ideal posture by Paul Chek. One image demonstrates ideal posture and the other is an example of poor posture:

Fig. 1	Fig. 2
Good Posture	**Poor Posture**

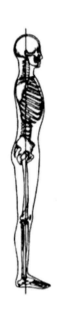 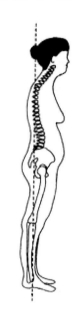

Source: Paul Chek Literature

That state of muscular and skeletal balance, which protects the supporting structures of the body against injury or progressive deformity, irrespective of the attitude in which these structures are working or resting. It is during a state of ideal posture that the muscles will function most efficiently.

In ideal posture, a line extending down the side of the body should run through the ear lobe, transect the shoulder, hip and knee joints and fall just anterior to (in front of) the ankle bone (Figure 1).

POSTURE

WHY DEVELOP THE HABIT OF GOOD POSTURE?

Good Posture and Your Life

"A good stance and posture reflect a proper state of mind."

~ Morihei Ueshiba

Our posture can tell a story about us. It represents what we have been through and what we are currently going through. How we carry our body can say a lot about how we carry ourselves through life. In other words, if you walk hunched over and drag your feet, it would appear that life is dragging you down. And life should not be a drag! It is a special gift! Maintaining good posture represents that we are conquering gravity's power (resistance) each and every day. Thus, it signifies that we can tackle any resistance and negative habits with our heads held high. Remember, how you carry yourself has the power to change your life!

Good Posture and Practicality

Good posture signifies confidence. It is well known that confidence can be of great value in our lives. In all areas of life, people with confidence will almost always excel over those who lack it. A good posture shows that a person is in control of their body and life. And it is this sense of power or control that makes a confident person attractive to others. Here are just some examples of how maintaining an upright posture with confidence can prove to be advantageous in multiple areas of life:

ONE HABIT AT A TIME

- **Students:** Students entering the workforce after graduation are told to maintain good posture while they are being interviewed by a potential employer. This is because most employers would not choose a defensive and withdrawn person over an aspiring, confident individual. The confident individual shows that they are ready to take on any assigned responsibilities as they have a more competent appearance. A confident image conveys that they will make natural leaders and they will more likely take positive initiative in their work environment. A confident student is more attractive to employers.

- **Athletes:** A great athlete knows the importance of maintaining good posture and confidence when in competition. Coaches will often repeat to their athletes to keep their heads up, especially in team sports. This increases the athlete's awareness of their surroundings, namely where their teammates and opponents are, thereby, increasing their chances of success. As for confidence, this attribute results in athletes playing at the top of their game. And when an athlete is at the top of their game, success is sure to follow. A confident playmaker is always welcome on any team.

- **Salespeople:** Salespeople are always told to have an upright and open posture. Why? Well, it shows that they are confident in what they are selling and it gives them a more trustworthy image. An upright posture shows that they are more attentive and listening to their customer's needs. Therefore, a salesperson with great confidence will outsell the one without. A successful salesperson brings increased profits and would be welcomed by any company.

Good Posture and Energy

"Upright Posture is the most efficient"

~ Moshe Feldenkrais

Here on earth, gravity is a natural force that we are constantly subjected to. In order to overcome this incessant battle, our bodies need energy. It is easy to overlook this phenomenon but every time you sit, stand, move, etc., your body uses energy. While you are in a standing position, hundreds of muscles are working to hold you up. You might not feel these muscles working initially, but ask anyone who has to stand all day at work and I am sure they will tell you how tiresome it can be. In good posture, the force of gravity is dispersed more efficiently throughout the musculo-skeletal system. In contrast, with poor posture the load is not distributed efficiently causing many muscles to overwork. This leads to an unnecessary increase in energy expenditure. In other words, poor posture will continually deplete your energy throughout the day.

Good Posture and Stress

A body in poor posture is a body under constant stress. The most important thing you can do to improve your health and vitality is to reduce the amount of overall stress in your life. Poor posture causes unnecessary stress to be placed on you, increasing your chances of suffering from pain and/or injury. The excess stress on the spine, joints and muscles causes a lot of people to live with unwanted inflammation and pain. Billions of dollars are spent (and wasted) annually on pharmaceuticals, surgery and various other types of treatments to alleviate the painful symptoms caused by poor posture. The problem with many treatments and drugs is that they do not solve the root cause of the pain. If a person's pain is caused by the habit of poor posture, then this is where the healing or correction should be focused.

Good Posture and Your Body

"Keeping your body healthy is an expression of gratitude to the whole cosmos - the trees, the clouds, everything."

~ Thich Nhat Hanh

Without a doubt, the human body is a wondrous part of our being. If you deeply study and think about all the complexities within the body's structure, you will understand that it is truly a masterpiece. It is absolutely one of the most marvellous gifts you have been given by the Creator of the universe. And because you are only given one body in this lifetime, it would be wise to keep it vital and strong. The habit of good posture is one of the best ways you can maintain this wonderful gift. Again, as the above quote states, by keeping your body healthy, you send a message to the Universe that you are grateful for this gift. (Gratefulness will be discussed in further detail in chapter 8)

POSTURE

Fig. 3

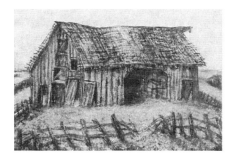

Watercolour by Howard Garrison

Fig. 4

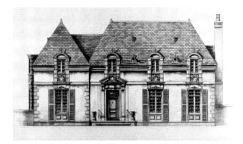

www.beaudaniels.com

    Your body is a temporary home or should even be considered as a temple for your soul and mind. If there was word of a hurricane about to strike your area, which of the houses shown above would you choose to take shelter in – Figure 3 (poor posture) or Figure 4 (good posture)? Which house would you feel more confident in during the storm? Which house is more attractive? The answer should be quite obvious.

ONE HABIT AT A TIME

Fig. 5

AGING EFFECTS OF POOR POSTURE

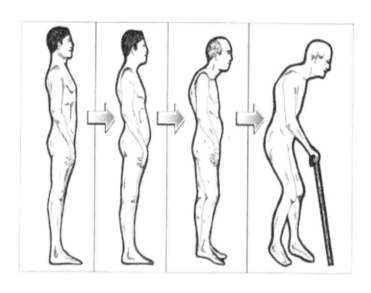

Source: www.chicagosportsmedicine.com

Figure 5 illustrates how the aging body slowly loses the battle with gravity when you do not maintain good posture. You must understand that even though aging can be accelerated by poor posture, poor posture is not the result of aging. Poor posture, for the most part, is a by-product of the accumulation of poor habits. It is the lack of practicing the habit of good posture that causes poor posture. The good news is that poor posture can be altered at any time. And even though aging cannot be prevented, maintaining good posture will aid the body in aging gracefully. Therefore, if you wish to age gracefully, it is your responsibility to develop the habit of good posture.

POSTURE

The Benefits of Good Posture

Remember, good posture signifies youth, strength, and vitality. Here is a list of some benefits of having good posture:

1. A proper ribcage position leads to improved breathing quality (the next chapter describes all of the benefits of high-quality breathing)

2. Muscular and skeletal balance leads to a reduced amount of stress on the spine, joints and muscles; since stress decreases energy, a reduced amount of stress would lead to an increase in energy

3. Less stress means less wear and tear on the body; this decreases the chances of injury, inflammation and arthritis

4. Correct spinal position allows the organs of the body to function optimally; this is because each organ is controlled by the nervous system which runs through the spine; each segment of the spine has different nerves running through it to a corresponding organ; in poor posture, these nerves can become compressed resulting in a lack of bioelectric energy flow; it is similar to having someone step on a hose while watering the lawn or on a vacuum hose while vacuuming; having a good posture decompresses all the nerves of the nervous system and allows for optimal neural output or nerve signal impulses to organs, muscles, etc.; please keep in mind that the word '*organ*' encompasses many bodily functions and systems; for instance, the digestive system, hormonal system, lymphatic (detoxification) system, circulatory system, eyes (vision), skin, and much more

5. When the spine, joints, and muscles are in their proper positions, there are no blockages in blood and energy flow thus you will have great circulation; with great circulation and neural output there is less chance of muscle cramping, fatigue, tingling, and numbness

6. Good posture can make you feel and appear more confident; confidence is a very attractive attribute

7. And much more; if you want continued health, longevity, and to age gracefully then you must learn and practice the habit of good posture

HOW TO DEVELOP THE HABIT OF GOOD POSTURE

Focus On the Good

"Inside of me there are two dogs. One of the dogs is mean and evil. The other dog is good. The mean dog fights the good dog, all of the time." When asked which dog wins, he reflected for a moment and replied
"The one I feed the most."

~ Wisdom attributed to an old Native American elder

It is critical to understand that poor posture is a habit and with practice, habits can be changed! The best way to change a habit is to consciously choose its opposite. For instance, if you have the habit of poor posture, do not focus on breaking the habit. Instead, focus on building its opposite – good posture. Basically, focus on what you want and do not focus on what you do not want.

This is an important principle of the law of attraction. What we focus on grows or expands because we are giving (feeding) it energy. Therefore, focus on (or feed) the habit you wish to develop and neglect (starve) the habit you wish to rid. For example, when the Habit Watch beeps, you are checking to see if you are or are not practicing the habit of good posture. You are not checking to see if you have poor posture. Please, it is imperative that you understand the difference between the two because it is essential for habit development. To increase your chances of success, you must use this technique of "focusing on the good" while developing any new habit.

Creating the Habit of Good Posture

"Unless some misfortune has made it impossible, everyone can have good posture."

~ Loretta Young

To develop the habit of good posture, set your Habit Watch to do a single beep (or vibration*) every 15, 30, or 60 minutes. Whenever the Habit Watch beeps, check and see if you are practicing the habit of good posture. If you are, great! Keep it up and give yourself a pat on the back. If you are not practicing the habit of good posture, then start doing so right away.

It is crucial that you do not get upset with yourself if you are not practicing the habit. At 15 minute intervals you will have checked your posture 4 times in one hour and 40 times in 10 hours. Therefore, even if you found yourself not practicing good posture all of those times, you have still readjusted your postural position 40 times. This is, in and of itself, a new habit. And you are well on your way to mastering the habit of good posture.

To master a habit, it must be practiced for at least 30 consecutive days. However, it may take longer for some individuals so do not get discouraged; take more time if you need it. How do you know when you have mastered a habit? You know you have mastered a habit when you find yourself practicing it at least 80% of the time. Only move on to the development of the next habit when you have mastered this one. It is essential that you do this if you want lasting results.

Figure 6 is an example of sitting with poor posture and Figure 7 shows how to practice the habit of good posture in a sitting position. (Figure 6 is far too common)

Fig.6   *Fig. 7*

Poor Posture   Good Posture

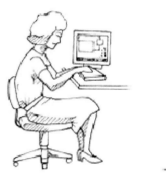
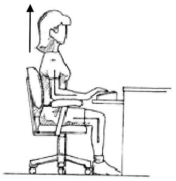

Source: Paul Chek Literature

POSTURE

Explanation of Figure 7: Start by placing your head over the center of your ribcage. This helps to relax the neck muscles. Notice the arrow behind the head is pointing upward. By lifting the crown of the head toward the ceiling or sky it lengthens the spine. Try it. Can you feel your spine lengthen? How does that feel? Your shoulders and arms are hanging directly over the middle of your ribcage. This further relaxes the neck muscles. Notice how the chest (ribcage) is lifted and positioned slightly in front of the head. Remember, upright posture does not mean to be stiff. On the contrary, it means to relax. So play around with the positioning of your body until you have found a good upright posture that you feel relaxed in. Please know that this may take some time. At first, upright posture will probably feel strenuous or uncomfortable, but the more you practice, the easier it will be to maintain. These points also apply to standing posture.

* Notes: The vibration alarm feature is a great option for the hearing impaired and for anyone who works in a noisy or noise sensitive environment.

Emotionalize the Habit

If properly guided, '*emotion*' can be a powerful tool in developing a habit. I call this process emotionalizing a habit. I have assigned a specific emotion to each habit in this book to aid in its development. I have carefully selected an emotion that I believe best compliments each habit. For the habit of good posture, I chose confidence as the supporting emotion. Confidence is a great foundational emotion for it will help you to succeed in all your endeavours and in the development of any habit. When you hear the Habit Watch beep, I want you to adjust your posture (if necessary), and FEEL CONFIDENT when doing so.

What if you are not a confident person? You might not be a confident person but I am sure we all know, to some degree, how it feels to be confident. Confidence is a state of mind or of being. It is similar to posture. You might have poor posture at this moment but if you keep self-correcting each time the Habit Watch beeps, you will soon find yourself with good posture.

As you now know, your posture can be readjusted and eventually reshaped. Well, it is no different with your state of mind (or mood). Your state of being can be readjusted and reshaped too. The more times you adjust your state of mind to feel confident, the easier it becomes to do so and eventually, it will become a natural way of being. In fact, with this simple method (Habit Watch), anything you desire can become a natural trait in your life. Isn't that amazing news? I hope you are excited!

Summary of Creating the Habit of Good Posture

- Focus on developing the new habit instead of focusing on breaking the old habit

- Set the Habit Watch to beep once every 15, 30, or 60 minutes

- When the Habit Watch beeps, check your posture

- If you are not in an upright position adjust your posture

- Try to be relaxed in your upright posture (not stiff)

POSTURE

- Feel a sense of confidence in your good postural position

- To master the habit practice it for at least 30 days

- You have mastered the habit when you catch yourself practicing it at least 80% of the time

CONCLUSION

Going the Extra Mile with the Habit of Good Posture

There are a number of ways in which a person may correct their posture. I believe one of the best approaches to postural correction is the one used by a C.H.E.K. practitioner as follows:

1 - EVALUATION
2 - PROGRAM DESIGN
3 - PROGRAM INSTRUCTION
4 - PROGRAM PROGRESSION

Step 1 – A thorough evaluation or assessment of the individual's current posture. Spinal curves, joints, and muscles range of motion should also be assessed. And much more!

Step 2 – A plan of correction will be devised based on the information collected from the assessment. The program includes strengthening, stretching and mobilization exercises. It may also include some supplementary bodywork (Massage Therapy, Feldenkrais, and

ONE HABIT AT A TIME

Acupuncture etc.), nutrition and lifestyle recommendations.

Step 3 – The program is then taught to the individual for proper implementation.

Step 4 – A re-evaluation is done after completing the correction program for the number of weeks and times specified. From there, a new program is designed to further progress the individual toward their goal(s).

If you want more information on C.H.E.K. practitioners or you would like to locate one in your area, please visit: www.chekinstitute.com.

The following are some more great resources for improving posture are listed below:

- Acupuncture
- Chiropractic
- Feldenkrais Method
- Neuro-Muscular Therapy
- Physical Therapy
- Rolfing
- Somatics
- Trigger Point Therapy
- Ergonomics
- Alexander Technique
- Cranio Sacral Therapy
- Hellerwork
- Osteopathy
- Qi Gong
- Shiatsu
- Tai chi
- Yoga

Note: Be sure to choose the right person to work with you. Always check reliable sources to see if the practitioner has a good reputation.

To get your Habit Watch or for more information and tools on developing the habit of good posture, please visit: **www.habitwatch.ca**.

POSTURE

Stand Tall!

Congratulations! You are NOW ready to use the Habit Watch to develop the habit of good posture. It is time for you to stand tall and walk with your head held high! It is time for you to be confident and attract all you desire in your life! And finally, it is time for you to be in control of your life and LIVE powerfully!

Habit 1 - Maintain a good upright posture and feel confident doing so.

After 30 consecutive days of mastering the habit of good posture, you will be ready to develop the habit of high-quality breathing.

2

Breathe

THE HABIT OF HIGH-QUALITY BREATHING

"Breathe. Let go. And remind yourself that this very moment is the only one you know you have for sure."

~ Oprah Winfrey

I want you to try a little experiment. You are going to take a deep breath in two different positions. In the first position, you will purposely slouch. In other words, round your shoulders, hunch your upper back and slide your head forward (See Figure 9). In the second position, you will consciously practice the habit you learned in the previous chapter – the habit of good posture (See figure 8). Go ahead and try them both. In which position are you able to take a deeper breath? After completing this simple experiment, you should understand why it was important to learn the habit of good posture before learning the habit of high-quality breathing.

When you stay in a slouched position, the ribcage is both depressed and compressed. In this position, the ribcage cannot fully expand, making it difficult to completely fill the lungs and take an optimal breath. Therefore, for an optimal breath, the ribcage should be uplifted as it is when you are in a good postural position. This is just added proof of the importance of having good posture as a fundamental habit.

As we all know, breathing is a necessity. Everyone must continuously breathe in order to stay alive, mainly because the brain cannot survive long without oxygen. For this reason, the body breathes instinctively and automatically without the use of the conscious mind. This is most obvious during sleep. However, even though breathing is an automatic function of the body, it does not mean that it should be ignored. This is because there are several types of breathing patterns the body can adopt, some are positive and others are not. In this chapter, you will learn the difference between high-quality (positive) and low-quality (negative) breathing patterns and you will learn how to develop the habit of high-quality breathing.

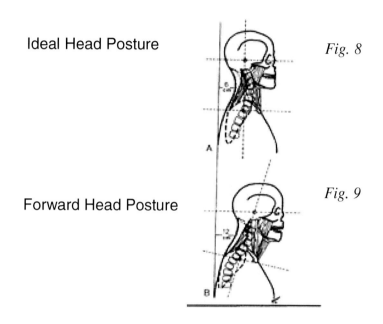

Ideal Head Posture — *Fig. 8*

Forward Head Posture — *Fig. 9*

Source: Paul Chek Literature

WHAT IS THE HABIT OF HIGH-QUALITY BREATHING?

High-quality Breathing & Low-quality Breathing

A simple definition of high-quality breathing is 'taking a full breath'. Some important aspects of high-quality breathing are; breathing from the nose, breathing from the diaphragm or abdomen, and taking less than 15 breaths per minute. Low-quality breathing means 'taking a shallow breath'. Mouth, chest-dominant, and rapid breathing are some traits of low-quality breathing. The subject of proper breathing is extensive. Therefore, just as I have done in the previous chapter, I have included a section at the end of this chapter titled 'going the extra mile with the habit of high-quality breathing' for any reader who wishes to learn more. Again, it is highly recommended that you indeed learn more about this habit.

WHY DEVELOP THE HABIT OF HIGH-QUALITY BREATHING?

High-quality Breathing and Your Life

"For breath is life, and if you breathe well you will live long on earth."

~ Sanskrit Proverb

Breathe in, breathe out, breathe in, and breathe out. This cyclical action of breathing in and out is what keeps you alive. Therefore, to become conscious of your breathing means to become conscious of life itself. By adopting the habit of high-quality breathing, you eventually take control of your breath. This control over your breath, leads to greater control over your stress levels, your mind, body, and emotions. And when you are in control of all of these things, you greatly increase your chances of living a long and healthy life.

High-quality Breathing and Practicality

We all know how good it feels when we are

relaxed. This is why so many people are willing to spend a lot of money on cottages, vacations, and spas, etc. I consider these things to be money well spent. However, I believe most people underestimate the power of breathing for relaxation. High-quality breathing can be done by anyone, at anytime or place, and best of all it's free! Remember, high-quality breathing and relaxation are synonymous with one another, whereas low-quality breathing and relaxation are not.

    Our breathing is automatic, thus we can breathe without being conscious of it. However, by doing this we lose control of our breathing quality. When we never focus our attention on something, we lose control of it. If you never think about your breathing, then how will you know the quality of your overall breathing? The fact is YOU WON'T! With the use of the Habit Watch, all of this will change. You will be more conscious of your breathing and you will have a lot more control over your breathing quality. As you may have noticed, *'control'* is a recurring theme because it is essential to the changing and developing of habits. If YOU are not in control of your life and habits, then who is? Here are some real life examples of why breathing and relaxation are so important:

- **Students:** Here is what happens when a student loses control due to the overwhelming pressure of exams. When a student is preparing for an exam, they study vigorously to achieve excellent test results. Often, students enter exams nervous and anxious. This leads to low-quality breathing. All they have studied suddenly escapes their mind. As the fear of failure escalates, their breath becomes increasingly rapid and shallow. This makes it even more difficult to remember the material, because their brain needs oxygen to function efficiently. This occurrence is more common than one might expect. That is why it is imperative to employ the habit of high-quality breathing and relaxation before, and during an exam. Relaxation will help you to reclaim control of your mind and memory. It will also give you the energy needed to study long hours and complete even the most lengthy of exams.

- **Athletes:** Athletes are well aware of the importance of relaxation. A boxer knows to remain relaxed during a fight. This enables the boxer to conserve energy for the later rounds. Tiger Woods is a great example of an athlete who is in control of himself during competition. His golf swing looks effortless. He knows not to tense up or he will lose control of it. His ability to stay relaxed, even in high-pressure situations, is what continually separates him from the rest of the field. In all sports, the ability to stay relaxed in high-pressure situations is what separates the champions from the ordinary athletes.

- **Salespeople:** If a salesperson does not stay relaxed, they will have a more difficult time making sales. If a sales person conveys any form of uneasiness, it can result in the loss of a sale. Why? Well, prospects can sense uneasiness and uneasiness usually implies that the salesperson does not believe in what they are selling. A salesperson must learn to remain relaxed even when there is a great deal of pressure to make the sale. A lot of people do not like high-pressure salespeople and neither do I. I

have walked away from products and services that I was already sold on because the salesperson pushed too far! If the salesperson believes in the value of the product or service they are selling, then there should be no need to get stressed about making sales. All that is required of them is to honestly convey their belief in the product or service and tell the prospect about all the great benefits.
Remember, a confident and relaxed salesperson will make plenty of sales.

High-quality Breathing and Energy

Tension usually leads to the expending of an unnecessary amount of energy. In contrast, when we are relaxed, we perform better and are more effective. Furthermore, a person that is breathing properly will take in more oxygen and will have more energy. Casinos are well aware of this fact as they purposely pump a lot of oxygen into the air, thereby causing the visitors to play longer! The casino sets the gaming odds in their favour so the longer people play, the more money the casino earns. It is a brilliant, yet sneaky ploy.

High-quality Breathing and Stress

"Stress is an ignorant state. It believes that everything is an emergency."

~ Natalie Goldberg

Stress has a huge impact on the way we breathe.

BREATHE

Different types of stressors can create several types of poor breathing patterns. Fear is one of the most common stressors that cause low-quality breathing. Our body's response to fear is instinctive. For example, when prey is being hunted by a predator, it will breathe shallowly so that it will not be heard. In such cases, a fear response is warranted. However, there are 2 types of fear – actual and presumed. Actual fear is when you are in a situation where your life is in real danger, i.e., being hunted by a lion! This is the type of fear that is necessary. Presumed fear is when you are not in any life threatening situation, i.e., stage fright. This type of fear is a stressor that we should reduce.

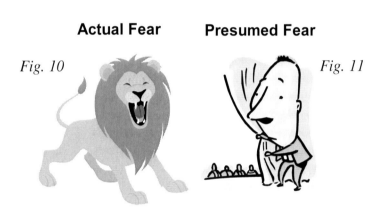

Fig. 10 — **Actual Fear** *Fig. 11* — **Presumed Fear**

"I quit being afraid when my first venture failed and the sky didn't fall down."
~Allen H. Neuharth

Confidence is a great character trait for reducing presumed fear as it has power over fear. This is another reason why I chose confidence as a fundamental emotion in chapter 1. Together with confidence, the habit of high-quality breathing will further reduce our presumed fear. High-quality breathing has a naturally calming effect on the nervous system, the mind, and the body. It is a great antidote for stress and anxiety. When a person is feeling any form of uneasiness, it is a common suggestion to take a deep breath and relax. And it is often suggested because it works.

High-quality Breathing for Your Health

I mentioned earlier that a person who is highly stressed will consume an unnecessary amount of energy. Also, a person under stress usually has a low-quality of breath and these two factors are known contributors to disease. I have seen the word "disease" broken down numerous times as dis-ease, or in other words, a person not at ease. A person not at ease means that they are not relaxed and are indeed stressed. Relaxation and stress (disease) are opposites. You cannot be extremely relaxed and stressed at the same time. For this reason, it is my strong belief, that one of THE MOST SIGNIFICANT AGENTS for preventing and even reversing disease (stress) is the habit of high-quality breathing (and the relaxation that accompanies it). I promise that you will begin to feel your health improve the moment you start practicing the habit of high-quality breathing.

High-quality Breathing and Your Mind

"When the breath wanders the mind also is unsteady. But when the breath is calmed the mind too will be still, and the yogi achieves long life. Therefore, one should learn to control the breath."

~ Svatmarama, *Hatha Yoga Pradipika*

BREATHE

The habit of high-quality breathing strongly prepares you for the development of the habits in part II – Three Essential Habits for the Mind. The breath is used in meditation to calm and take control of the mind. The mind is capable of thinking many thoughts in succession for long periods of time. However, ceaseless thinking, of the unconscious kind, should be avoided because it is very draining to your energy stores given that thought is energy. In other words, every thought that is released takes energy from you. Therefore, if the mind is allowed to run wild, it will be a great stressor in your life. And I assure you that this is a common problem for just about everyone in this world. Remember, focusing on the breath will slow the amount of thoughts (energy) released by the mind and this will reduce the stress caused by ceaseless thinking.

High-quality Breathing and Your Body

Remember, high-quality breathing is another fantastic way to show gratitude to your body. You should be grateful because every breath you take keeps you alive. Essentially, when you breathe in, you breathe in life – you breathe in energy. Oxygen is our main source of energy production. In fact, it is more important to energy production than food or water. You could survive without food and water for several days but you cannot survive without oxygen for more than 5 minutes!   As you can see, breathing has a much greater impact on our bodies than most people realize. For this reason, I find it odd that there is so much more emphasis on eating proper food diets than developing high-quality breathing. I am not saying that proper food diets are not important but rather that breathing quality is too often neglected or overlooked.

ONE HABIT AT A TIME

There is an old saying, *"if you don't use it, you will lose it"*. When your breathing quality is neglected, it will slowly diminish over time. Furthermore, the lower your breathing quality is, the more susceptive you will be to stress, disease and aging. Remember, a person that is continuously stressed will age more quickly than if they were habitually relaxed. Therefore, it is your responsibility to develop the habit of high-quality breathing in order to combat stress, prevent disease and age gracefully.

The Benefits of High-Quality Breathing

Here is a list of some benefits that you can look forward to by maintaining high-quality breathing:

1. The body needs oxygen to function optimally and to assist in the generation of its energy; therefore, an increased amount of oxygen leads to having more energy to operate all of the body's systems (nervous, digestive, lymphatic, and so on)

2. Oxygen and energy support and strengthen the immune system; this leads to getting fewer flu viruses, colds, and other common sicknesses; in addition, common viruses and bacteria cannot survive in oxygenated environments

3. Oxygen and relaxation reduce the overall amount of stress on the body and its systems; lowering negative stress decreases the chances of disease; Nobel Prize winner Otto Warburg is a scientist who discovered that if a cell loses 60% of its oxygen it becomes cancerous

BREATHE

4. Less stress and more oxygen lead to less body fat; too much stress will lead to the over-production and release of cortisol, a stress hormone that is linked to the storing of body fat; also, oxygen increases metabolism function and mobilizes toxins from the body; toxins are stored in adipose (body fat) tissue, therefore, fewer toxins in the body means less body fat is needed

5. Oxygen and relaxation support and help the detoxification system to remove harmful toxins from the body; as a result, this further reduces the amount of body fat needed to store these dangerous toxins

6. With high-quality, the diaphragm moves upward and downward massaging the digestive organs, this improves digestion and peristalsis

7. Relaxation reduces the stress on the heart and this leads to a balance in blood pressure

8. An increase in the oxygen supply will improve mental clarity and memory

9. And much more; if you want continued health, longevity, and to age gracefully then you must also learn and practice the habit of high-quality breathing

Source:
(http://www.bodymindspiritguide.com/printFriendly.cfm?articleID=1719)

HOW TO DEVELOP THE HABIT OF HIGH-QUALITY BREATHING

Creating the Habit of High-Quality Breathing

Here are the 3 main differences between low-quality and high-quality breathing:

	Low-Quality Breathing	**High-Quality Breathing**
1.	Mouth breathing	Nasal breathing
2.	Chest-dominant (intercostal breathing) Shallow breaths (25-50% lung capacity)	Abdominal (diaphragmatic breathing) Full breaths (75-80% lung capacity)
3.	Rapid and irregular More than 15 breaths per minute	Slow & regular Less than 15 breaths per minute

Breathing from the nose is far better than breathing from the mouth. The nose is able to warm or cool the air coming into the lungs. The nose also acts as a filter for unwanted air particles. In addition, nose breathing opens lower regions of our lungs allowing us to take deeper breaths. It is common for people with forward head posture to breathe in from their mouth. When someone has forward head posture, it is easier to breathe in from the mouth because the nasal passage is partially restricted. (Refer back to figure 9)   This is another example of how posture can affect breathing. Therefore, the first part of high-quality breathing is to ensure that you are in a good

BREATHE

postural position and then breathe through the nose.

     The second part of high-quality breathing is abdominal breathing. Abdominal breathing is much more efficient than chest-dominant breathing. Abdominal breathing means using the diaphragm to breathe. The diaphragm is a muscle between the digestive organs and the lungs. On inhalation, the diaphragm moves downward, compressing the digestive system and causing the abdominal wall (belly) to protrude. This also allows the lungs to be fully filled with air (oxygen). On exhalation, the diaphragm moves upward, compressing the lungs and expelling the air (carbon dioxide). (Figure 12 shows the mechanics of high-quality breathing) Diaphragmatic breathing allows air to reach deeper parts of the lungs and aids in a more efficient expulsion of carbon dioxide than chest-dominant breathing. Please note that the chest may be used to breathe in conjunction with the diaphragm but breathing with the chest alone (chest-dominant breathing) should be avoided.

     An optimal breath should also be slow and regular. To determine your breathing rate just time yourself and see how many breaths you take in one minute. If you breathe more than 15 times in one minute, then you need to slow it down. Taking deeper breaths from nose and abdominal breathing should help lower the number of breaths you take in a minute. Regularity of breath is also important. Your inhalation time frame should be even with your exhalation time frame. Do not favour one over the other. The inhalation phase should flow smoothly into the exhalation phase and the exhalation phase should also flow smoothly into the inhalation phase. So remember, when breathing, slow and steady wins the race. The third part of high-quality breathing is to breathe slowly and smoothly.

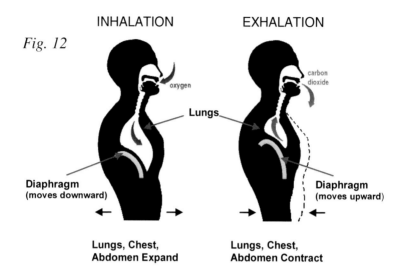

Fig. 12

High-quality Breathing and Hydration

    When you begin to practice the habit of high-quality breathing, you will probably notice yourself getting dehydrated more quickly. This is simply because the human body consumes water for the breathing process. This has not been mentioned previously, but dehydration is another factor that can contribute to low-quality breathing. When the body is dehydrated, it will instinctively breathe shallower to conserve water. Therefore, in order to maintain high-quality breathing, you must stay well hydrated. This advice is not to be taken lightly. I could have easily dedicated an entire chapter on maintaining proper hydration (as a habit).

    As we all know, water is an essential nutrient for our well being. Approximately 75% of our body composition is water. Please, stop and think about that for a moment. Three quarters of our body is water! Isn't that amazing? We are a walking pool of water! However, the water does not just stay still. It is incessantly utilized by our body to perform billions of functions that are necessary for our continued existence.

Most people know the importance of water, yet dehydration continues to be a common issue in our world. With our hectic lifestyles, we often forget to stop and drink a glass of water. To make matters worse, persuasive advertising has influenced many people to drink other products as a replacement for water. A lot of these beverages contain substances such as caffeine, which are dehydrants. In addition, many products are often loaded with processed sugars, artificial colours/flavours, and numerous other ingredients that are hazardous to our health. Please remember, water is the best source of fluid we can drink for optimal hydration and there are no substitutes!

Here are 5 tips for optimal hydration:

Tip 1 – In total, you should drink half of your body weight in ounces and even more in hot climates or when exercising. For example, a 150 lb person should drink at least 75 ounces of water per day. (Please keep in mind that these are just general guidelines.)

Tip 2 – Drink clean spring or purified water. Stay away from tap water as it contains many contaminants. Also, some water purifiers can deplete the water of its natural minerals. Adding a very small pinch of unprocessed sea salt is a good idea as it contains over 80 trace minerals. What's more, sea salt has the ability to prevent frequent urination along with numerous other health benefits.

ONE HABIT AT A TIME

Tip 3 – It is crucial to ensure that water is accessible to you at all times. Carry a bottle of water to places that might not have clean water available. When possible, use glass bottles instead of plastic. Water erodes plastic and many harmful chemicals are then mixed into the water. Yuck!

Tip 4 – Commit this old Tibetan saying to memory, "Drink your food and chew your water." Too many people quickly gulp down everything that enters their mouth. Take the time to swish the water around in your mouth where it will combine with your saliva. Saliva contains digestive enzymes that will assist in the assimilation of water (and food). Remember, digestion and hydration begins in the mouth!

Tip 5 – Drink water at room temperature (or slightly above) because it is most easily digestible for your body. Cold water just sits in the stomach and waits to be warmed before digestion. When you chug cold water, the stomach will get bloated. This is to prevent anymore cold water from entering the stomach. If you do drink cold water, ensure to swirl the water around in your mouth before you swallow. This swirling will warm the water to a more easily digestible temperature and your stomach will thank you for doing so.

Follow these tips and you will be on your way to optimal hydration.

Source: "How to Eat, Move and Be Healthy" by Paul Chek

BREATHE

Emotionalize the Habit

"Sometimes the most important thing in a whole day is the rest we take between two deep breaths".

~ Etty Hillesum

In chapter one, I described how emotion can be positively harnessed to support the development of a habit. For the habit of high-quality breathing, I have chosen the feeling of relaxation as the supporting emotion. When you practice the habit of high-quality breathing, I want you to notice and focus on how relaxing it feels. Remember, what you focus on expands. If you focus on your stressors, you will become more stressed, but if instead, you focus on relaxing, you will relax. It is that simple! Also, you must understand that no matter how stressed you are, the moment you focus on high-quality breathing and relaxing, you will begin to relax. This might sound too good to be true, right? Well, just give a try and see for yourself.

Once again, when practicing the habit of high-quality breathing, I want you to feel an overall sense of relaxation. Start by relaxing any muscles that may feel tense. Relax your mind from stressful thoughts. Relax anything that is causing you stress or tension. There may be times, when the Habit Watch beeps, that you will find yourself in the middle of a stressful situation. It could be that you are in an argument at home or trying to meet a deadline for work. Whatever the case, it is at these stressful moments that high-quality breathing and relaxation are needed most.

Can someone really have control over how they feel? What if something terrible happens to you, how can you relax then? Human beings can only control 3 things;

their thoughts, feelings, and actions. In later chapters, I will discuss thoughts and actions, but for now, let's take a look at controlling emotion (how you feel). Emotion is an inward feeling. How you feel comes from within your being. You have the ability to choose how you want to feel at any given moment.

The problem is that most people allow external circumstances to dictate how they feel. An example of this is apparent in the common expression "I will be happy when…such and such happens". However, you do not have to wait for anything to happen in order for you to be happy. Happiness (or any emotion) is a state of being and we have the power to decide our state of being at all times. This power is a gift from the Universe.

Two people viewing the same event could have a completely different emotional response. This is extremely evident when listening to all the critics' reviews at the end of a movie. Likewise, two similar events can occur in your life and you can have a completely different emotional response for each situation. For example, one day while driving, you get cut off by a car and you go into a rage. Another day it happens again and it does not even faze you. Maybe, you even laugh about the situation. The event or circumstance was the same but your REACTION (emotional response) was different.

Therefore, I am asking you to stop giving your power away to circumstance. Do not allow anyone, anything, or any event to dictate how you are feeling in any given moment. Never say to someone that 'they make you angry' because this is not true. The truth is that you ALLOW them to make you angry. How you think, feel, and act is your responsibility. If you wish to be angry (or any other emotion), then be angry, but know that it is you who are choosing to be so.

Furthermore, you must know that you cannot control circumstance. Likewise, you cannot control how others think, feel, and act. What others think, feel, and do is their choice and responsibility. Remember, trying to control circumstance (or other people) leads to STRESS. Therefore, focus on controlling yourself and RELAX.

Summary of Creating the Habit of High-Quality Breathing

- Focus on developing the new habit instead of focusing on breaking the old habit

- Set the Habit Watch to beep once every 15, 30, or 60 minutes

- When the Habit Watch goes off, make sure that you are in a good postural position first and then examine your breathing quality

- Breathe through your nose

- Use your diaphragm (Note, when you inhale your belly expands or moves outward and when you exhale your belly moves inward toward your spine; this is important because a lot of people breathe backwards! I did not mention this earlier, but a backward breathing pattern is another form of low-quality breathing.)

- Breathe slowly

- Maintain optimal hydration

ONE HABIT AT A TIME

- Feel a sense of relaxation as you breathe

- To master the habit practice it for at least 30 days

- You have mastered the habit when you catch yourself practicing it at least 80% of the time

CONCLUSION

Going the Extra Mile with the Habit of High-Quality Breathing

If you find breathing interesting and would like to learn more, I have listed some breathing techniques and resources below.

Here are some of the many types of breathing techniques that one can practice:

- Alternate Nostril Breathing
- Piston Breathing
- Deep Breathing
- Relaxation Breathing
- Imaginative Breathing
- The Rolling Breath
- Meditative Breathing
- Zone Breathing

Here are some great resources that integrate the breath with posture and movement:

- Alexander Technique

BREATHE

- C.H.E.K. Holistic Lifestyle Coaching
- Feldenkrais Method
- Martial Arts
- Qi Gong
- Tai Chi
- Yoga

For more tools and information on developing the habit of high-quality breathing, please visit: **www.habitwatch.ca**.

Breathe. Let Go!

Congratulations! You are NOW ready to use the Habit Watch to develop the habit of high-quality breathing. It is time for you to lead a more relaxed and productive life. It is time for you to let go of stress and set yourself free of it for good! And finally, it is time for you to be in control of your emotions and FEEL the way you want!

Habit 2 - Maintain a high-quality of breathing and feel relaxed doing so.

After 30 consecutive days of mastering the habit of high-quality, breathing you will be ready to develop the habit of smiling.

3

Smile

THE HABIT OF SMILING

"A smile is the universal welcome."

~ Max Eastman

     I cheerfully welcome you to the third and final habit of part I – the habit of smiling. For many reasons, the habit of smiling compliments and adds a nice touch to the previous habits. For instance, when you walk around with good posture and confidence, it can often be mistaken as conceit if it is not accompanied by a cheerful smile. On the flip side, adding a genuine smile to your posture communicates that you are an open and caring individual. A smile will make your confidence more amiable because it has the power to turn an arrogant image into a pleasant or humble one.
     Furthermore, you will more likely see a smile on a

person who is relaxed than one who is stressed. This is because it is difficult to be really stressed and have a genuine smile at the same time. A confident and relaxed person will smile more often and with greater ease because all of these feelings are positive and congruent. In other words, confidence, relaxation, and cheerfulness all feel good. Here is an example of how these three habits flow into each other. If you had to give a presentation, you would first want to be confident. Once you are confident in what you will be presenting, you will naturally feel and be more relaxed. And finally, relaxation allows you to enjoy the process of presenting.

      Now, I ask you to please close your eyes and think of someone you know who often smiles at you. Hold the image of that person smiling in your mind. How does this image of their smiling make you feel? Now, on the contrary, think of someone you know who never smiles and always frowns at you. How does this image make you feel? Which one of these 2 people are more welcoming?

      This simple exercise demonstrates the power of a smile. You can be a wonderful person but no one, whom you first meet, will ever know it if you hide behind a sulking or expressionless face. When you wear a smile, you are welcoming people into your life. In fact, a smile communicates many messages. It says 'hi, how are you?', 'I am willing to engage in conversation', 'I am willing to help you', 'I am friendly', 'I am interested in getting to know you better', 'I enjoy your presence', etc. As you can see, there are numerous positive communications that a single smile can express. In this chapter, you will learn all about the habit of smiling and the impact it can have on your life.

ONE HABIT AT A TIME

WHAT IS THE HABIT OF SMILING?

Smiling & Frowning

"A smile is the light in your window that tells others that there is a caring, sharing person inside."

~ Denis Waitley

      The habit of smiling is not just the physical lifting of the edges of your lips. It must be genuine and, to be genuine, it must come from within. A real smile is filled with cheerfulness, signifying that cheerfulness and smiling are inseparable. Cheerfulness is an inward state of being and a smile is the outward expression of this state of being. Therefore, to have the habit of smiling, you must be cheerful. In this chapter, frowning, sulking, or having an expressionless face are habits we will be aiming to avoid.
      Cheerfulness comes from within, not from without. Yet, most people tend to search for cheerfulness in people, places or things outside of themselves. I often hear people make such comments as; 'When I meet Mr. (or Ms.) Right, I will be happy', 'When I finish school and travel the world, then I will be happy', 'When I win the lottery, I will be happy' and so on. Maybe you will be happy when these things do come true, but why wait? You could be cheerful at anytime. Remember, these situations only draw out the happiness that is always there inside you.
      Looking for or relying on outside circumstances to feel good is a dangerous way of living. Why? It is one of the main reasons people become addicted to all sorts of substances and habits. The rush one gets from gambling, the high one feels from a drug, or the emotional pain that is

numbed by alcohol, are all common examples of substance abuse. These all give you a false sense of cheerfulness or feeling good. It is a temporary feeling that will soon subside and will leave you thirsting for more. Remember, authentic cheerfulness comes from your inner spirit and anything that emanates from the spirit is infinite (not temporary).

WHY DEVELOP THE HABIT OF SMILING?

Smiling and Your Life

"Anyone who has a continuous smile on his face conceals a toughness that is almost frightening."

~ Greta Garbo

How does a continuous smile conceal toughness? As mentioned in the previous chapters, the habits in this book are about taking control of your life. Posture, breathing and smiling are all physical traits but are very much internal traits too. For example, it takes a person of great character to maintain a good posture while confidently admitting to a mistake. In addition, it takes great character to breathe deeply and be relaxed when under immense pressure. And finally, it requires a tough character to smile and maintain a cheerful attitude in times of opposition, adversity or misfortune.

A persons' strength of character comes from within. Thus, to have a continuous smile on your face signifies having control over your inner state of being. And to take control of your life, you must be in control of your inner state of being. Remember, you can choose your inner state of being at any moment. If you focus on being confident, relaxed and/or joyous, you can become so immediately. You possess this power and you should never give it away to others or to circumstance. When you retain your power, you will become captain of your ship (life). (I will explain the concept of captaining your ship in further detail in the next chapter.)

Smiling and Practicality

A genuine smile is charismatic. It has a strong magnetic force that draws people toward you. Why is it so attractive? A smile tells everyone around you that you are feeling good and everyone loves feeling good. They want some of that positive energy that smiling gives off, so they can feel good too.

Smiling has the ability to change the mood of everyone in a room. I am sure you can think of at least one person in your life that has this ability. If not, think of how the mood changes the moment a smiling baby enters a room. I have seen people in the grumpiest of moods smile from ear to ear after spending just a few seconds with a baby. This further proves that a cheerful smile is one of the most contagious things in this world. So spread the positivity and smile. Below are some real life examples of how cheerfulness and smiling can improve your life:

- **Students:** Cheerfulness emanates a positive energy that can be felt by any interviewer. The moment a cheerful student walks into the interviewing room, the air becomes lighter. A smile has the power to light up an emotionally dark room and it can easily be the deciding factor between two, equally qualified interviewees. Any employer would love to welcome a positive force to their work team. Team work is a necessity in the workplace and a person who smiles shows that they are ready to be part of a team.

- **Business:** There is an old Chinese proverb that states *"Don't open a shop unless you like to smile."* Many vendors sell the exact same products or services, but it is the vendor with the most charisma that will be more successful. As previously mentioned, a cheerful smile is charismatic and it has a powerful magnetic force that will keep customers coming back to do business with you. Remember, people like to do business with people, not businesses. A smile shows that you, the vendor, are not just another business but, in fact, a person. At the same time, a smile shows that the customer is not just another customer but a unique person.

- **Salespeople:** When a salesperson is cheerful and smiling, they are giving off positive energy. The prospective buyer feels this energy and will naturally become more interested in the product/service being sold. Why? Cheerfulness conveys that the salesperson feels genuinely good about the product/service they are selling. And the customer usually assumes that it is because the product/service is improving the lives of all who have purchased it. Remember, the customer can sense (consciously or unconsciously) whether or not a salesperson believes in their product/service. Adding a cheerful smile to an already confident and relaxed demeanour, will improve your sales results even further.

ONE HABIT AT A TIME

Cheerfulness and Energy

"A merry heart goes all the day, A sad tires in a mile."

~ William Shakespeare

Have you ever noticed how much energy you have when you are cheerful? What do you do when you are cheerful? Do you smile? Do you walk with sort of a bounce in your step? Do you sing a song or whistle a tune? Do you dance? Many people do, as these are just some natural responses to being cheerful. It is as if there is an abundance of energy inside you that needs to be released or you will explode! This is how you could feel everyday of your life if you make cheerfulness a habit!

Cheerfulness and Stress

A simple formula to remember is 'less stress equals more energy'. Therefore, if you want to have an abundance of energy throughout each day, you have to learn to manage and reduce your stress. The good news is that every habit in this book is a stress reducing habit. In the previous chapter, you learned that stress and relaxation are opposites. Likewise, stress and cheerfulness are antagonistic. It is difficult to be cheerful (and/or relaxed) and be stressed at the same time. The opposite of cheerfulness is wretchedness, hopelessness, depression, etc. and these are stressful emotions that will zap your energy when you allow them to dominate your mood.

SMILE

Cheerfulness and Fear

"A cheerful frame of mind, reinforced by relaxation... is the medicine that puts all ghosts of fear on the run."

~ George Matthew Adams

Cheerfulness is another kryptonite for fear. With every habit you build in this book, your presumed fear becomes weaker and weaker. Presumed fear is usually anxiety, a nervousness about something that might happen in the future. However, I have and will continue to repeat this truth many times throughout this book; you can always choose your mood or inner state of being. And you choose this inner state of being in the present moment, not the future. Therefore, you are not going to give your power away to circumstance whether it is in the past, present, or future. Remember, you can always choose to be cheerful, RIGHT NOW, no matter what has happened in your past, what is happening in the present, or what you may think will happen in your future.

Cheerfulness and Your Health

"A laughter a day keeps the doctor away. Be ever cheerful in whatever difficult conditions you may be placed. A cheerless mind is a diseased mind. Cheerfulness will let you tap the power within you. It will turn failure into success."

~ Sri Swami Shivananada

I had a powerful dream not that long ago. In this dream, I envisioned a beautiful woman about 25 years of age. She had magnificent hair colour which I had never seen before. It was a reddish gold colour that shined so bright it seemed to glow. To add to the magnificence, her hair was long with lots of large locks. Then, I remember watching her approach me with an unforgettable smile and she said "Hi my name is Joy and I am an energy healer. I can balance anyone's chakras (any of several points of physical or spiritual energy in the human body according to yoga philosophy)". She then said "I have the ability to cure any disease; diabetes, cancer, depression or anything else, for that matter."

     At first, I thought she was just trying to sell me something, but as I continued to listen to her speak, I suddenly realized something. There was something extremely special about this whole experience. It wasn't what she said that made me come to this realization, but it was the way she had said it, as she spoke with such conviction and truth. Upon this realization I asked "What is your name again?", in case I had misheard the first time, and with her angelic smile she replied "Joy". Immediately after she said that, I experienced an overwhelming feeling of pure joy and I awoke from my dream with a huge smile upon my face. I thought to myself and said "Wow! What a great message! Joy has the ability to heal disease."

     It makes so much sense. To be joyful means to be full of joy and to be diseased means to not be at ease. When a person is not at ease, it means that they are troubled, depressed and so on. These traits are of the opposite nature of joyfulness. Naturally, I came to the conclusion that joy is another powerful agent to prevent and reverse disease. Therefore, if you want a life of health and vitality, you must choose to develop the habit of smiling and make joy your regular companion.

SMILE

(Note: Please keep in mind that joyfulness, cheerfulness, and merriness are all synonymous and they will be used interchangeably throughout the chapter.)

The Benefits of a Smile

"We shall never know all the good that a simple smile can do."

~ Mother Teresa

Here is a list of some benefits that you can anticipate by adopting the habit of smiling:

1. It is practically impossible to have a cheerful smile and feel stressed at the same time because they are opposites; therefore keep smiling and you will keep stress away

2. When you have a genuine smile, you naturally feel more relaxed; in the previous chapter, I gave a list of all the benefits for relaxation so you can view those again for a refresher (stronger immune system, balanced hormone levels, lower blood pressure, etc.)

3. Smiling releases chemicals in your brain and body that act as natural drugs; if you have any pain, smiling can release natural endorphins (pain killers) to ease your pain; also, smiling can increase serotonin levels which are neurotransmitters that will make you feel good (and there are countless benefits to feeling good)

4. A lot people are worried about their appearance; this is why the cosmetics, fashion and weight loss industries make

ONE HABIT AT A TIME

billions of dollars; remember, a smile is the fastest, easiest, and best way to increase your appearance; and it's free

5. Smiling increases our energy levels; and more importantly the energy it increases is positive; you will be more productive, more attractive, and more successful, among other things

6. And much more; if you want to cast away negative moods such as wretchedness, anxiousness, and depression, then you must develop the habit of having a cheerful smile

The Value of a Smile

"It costs nothing, but creates much. It enriches those who receive, without impoverishing those who give. It happens in a flash and the memory of it sometimes lasts forever. None are so rich they can get along without it, and none so poor but are richer for its benefits."

"It creates happiness in the home, fosters goodwill in a business, and is the countersign of friends. It is rest to the weary, daylight to the discouraged, sunshine to the sad, and natures best antidote for trouble."

"Yet it cannot be bought, begged, borrowed or stolen, for it is something that is no earthly good to anyone 'til it is given away. And if in the hurly-burly bustle of today's business world, some of the people you meet should be too tired to give you a smile, may we ask you to leave one of yours?"

"For nobody needs a smile so much, as those who have none left to give."

~ Dale Carnegie
("How to Win Friends and Influence People")

SMILE

HOW TO DEVELOP THE HABIT OF SMILING

Use the Law of Attraction

"Men (people) do not attract that which they want, but that which they are."

~ James Allen

It is imperative that you understand the concept of attraction. Wanting something and being something are two different things. How are they different? I will use the example of money to explain the difference. If I declare that "I want a billion dollars!", it is far less powerful than declaring "I am a billionaire!". The former is coming from without and the latter statement is coming from within.

Donald Trump is a well known billionaire who at one time had lost his fortune. However, even though Donald Trump went bankrupt, he managed to regain his fortune. How was he able to amass such a large fortune again when most people cannot even accomplish this extraordinary feat even once? The main reason is because he never stopped BEING a billionaire. He only lost his outward or tangible fortune but his inward fortune remained. Donald Trump's true fortune consists of certain principles which he lives by, that attracted the riches he had lost back to him.

To state that you want a billion dollars (or happiness, etc.) is fine. But that alone will not get you there. You have to first be that which you desire, then you will begin to attract it. If you want a billion dollars, then study billionaires. How do they think? How do they act? What are some of the common character traits amongst billionaires? What are their HABITS? Once you have gathered an understanding of what it is to be a billionaire, start being one immediately, not just for one day, but every day for the rest of your life.

Declare Ownership and Take Responsibility

Lay not up for yourselves treasures upon earth, where moth and rust doth corrupt, and where thieves break through and steal. But lay up for yourselves treasures in heaven, where neither moth nor rust doth corrupt, and where thieves do not break through nor steal. For where your treasure is, there will your heart be also.

~ King James Bible (Matthew 6:19-21)

The words of the bible verse above was Jesus' way of communicating the difference between our outwardly possessions and our inwardly possessions. Outwardly possessions can be destroyed and stolen but our inwardly possessions cannot. Again, I will use the Donald Trump example. His outwardly possessions at one time were lost but the riches he possessed from within were not. He thought, felt and acted like a billionaire. And as long as he continues to think, feel and act like a billionaire, he will always retain his riches.

On the contrary, a person who earns riches through circumstance, chance or luck will more likely lose them. In fact, a common occurrence amongst people who win the lottery is that it is lost within a few years. This is because the money they possessed did not come from an inner way of being. They did not build or weave the characteristics or habits that are necessary to become a multi-millionaire. In truth, they were outwardly rich and inwardly poor.

Likewise, cheerfulness that comes from within can never be destroyed or stolen. On the contrary, cheerfulness based on an external circumstance can easily disappear. Therefore, do not wait for good things to happen to you in order to be cheerful. Be cheerful first and then you will attract the things that resonate and accentuate your cheerfulness. Unfortunately, most people have this concept backwards.

For some reason, most people need an excuse to be cheerful. People often ask me "Oh, what are you so happy about?" In their mind, something good must have happened in order for me to be happy. Again, this is backward or inaccurate thinking. I (or anyone) can feel good at any time, regardless of what has happened, is happening, or proposed to happen.

Confidence, relaxation, and cheerfulness all come from within. You OWN them! They are yours at any time and forever. All you need to do is learn to draw them out. The more often you draw them out, the easier it gets to do so. It is similar to working a muscle you rarely use. At first it will be weak, but use it continuously and it will get stronger and stronger. So, the first step to creating the habit of smiling is to declare ownership of your cheerfulness (or any other feeling, thought and action)

Ownership does come with responsibility, however. Now that you own your way of being, it is your responsibility to maintain it. For instance, if an outer circumstance occurs and it makes you angry, you have actually allowed this to happen (not the circumstance, but the feeling of anger). Remember, nothing (or no one) can make you feel a certain way without your consent. Therefore, it is solely your responsibility to maintain your cheerfulness. The second step to creating the habit of smiling is by taking responsibility of your thoughts, feelings, and actions because they create who you are (character traits, habits, and your way of being, etc.).

Creating the Habit of Smiling

"Smiling actually produces a biological effect in your body. It sends chemicals racing around your body and actually lifts your spirits. Try this today. Then, every day this week, smile five times a day for no good reason. Do it sitting in traffic. Do it standing in the shower. Do it walking down the street, or working at your desk. For no good reason, just break into a smile. Watch your mood change, even though nothing in your exterior has shifted."

~ Neale Donald Walsh

Set the habit watch to beep every 15, 30, or 60 minutes. Beep! Beep! Are you smiling? No, then start smiling. Yes, keep smiling. With the use of the Habit Watch it really is that simple and I love simplicity!

A Helpful Perspective

"I am determined to be cheerful and happy in whatever situation I may find myself. For I have learned that the greater part of our misery or unhappiness is determined not by our circumstances but by our disposition."

~ Martha Washington

It is your choice as to whether you see the glass as

half-empty or half-full. In order to maintain a cheerful attitude, you need to adopt the "glass half-full" perspective. You need to learn to look at the bright side of every situation. Maintaining this perspective can be extremely difficult, but practice it long enough and it will become second nature. Do not allow tough circumstances to bring you down. Learn to rise above challenging times. Try to think of difficult circumstances as opportunities to strengthen your character. If you can be cheerful during life's storms, imagine how cheerful you will be during the good times. Use the power of focus. Practice holding this perspective long enough and you will begin to see good times more often.

Emotionalize the Habit

> *"Sometimes your joy is the source of your smile, but sometimes your smile can be the source of your joy."*
>
> **~ Thich Nhat Hanh**

As previously mentioned, a genuine smile comes from within. Therefore, the power of a smile is measured by the amount of joy (or cheer) it expresses. The emotion of joy is believed to come from the 3rd chakra (1 of 7 major energy centers in the human being). The 3rd chakra is the area between the navel and the solar plexus (shown in figure 13). The colour of this energy center is yellow. If you wish to draw out joy from within, a great technique is to visualize this area shining bright like the sun (hence the name SOLAR plexus). This could explain why, like the sun, cheerful people brighten and warm up a room.

ONE HABIT AT A TIME

If worse comes to worse and you still do not feel like smiling, then you may need to use some other methods. One method is to smile first, and then see if this helps to draw out your joy from within. Another method that can be positively used to draw out your joy is to begin recognizing the POSITIVE people or things within your life that make you smile, like a specific person or pet, for example. There must be something in your life that makes you smile. Once you have figured out what makes you smile, use it as leverage to get you smiling. However, please keep in mind that this is only a temporary technique of using an outward means to draw out your inner joy. Eventually, you should be able to feel an abundance of joy emanating from within, whenever you choose to tune into it.

SOLAR PLEXUS CHAKRA

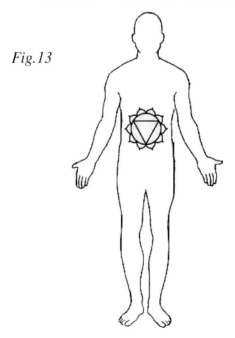

Fig.13

SMILE

Summary of Creating the Habit of Smiling

- Focus on developing the new habit instead of focusing on breaking the old habit

- Remember, you attract WHAT YOU ARE! So BE what you want to attract

- Claim ownership and take full responsibility over your thoughts, feelings and actions because they create who you are

- Set the Habit Watch to beep once every 15, 30, or 60 minutes

- When the Habit Watch goes off, check all previously learned habits and notice your facial expression

- If you are not smiling, change that by smiling with your whole being

- Maintain the "glass half-full" perspective and always look at the bright side of every situation

- Feel the joyfulness you possess emanating from within as you smile

- Visualize a small Sun shining from your solar plexus

- To master the habit practice it for at least 30 days

- You have mastered the habit when you catch yourself practicing it at least 80% of the time

CONCLUSION

Smile and Enjoy!

Congratulations! You are NOW ready to use the Habit Watch to develop the habit of smiling. It is time for you to smile with your whole being! It is time for you to rise above circumstance and be cheerful no matter what life brings! And finally, it is time for you to lead a more joyful life and to infect others with your joy!

Habit 3 - Maintain a cheerful attitude by using the habit of smiling.

After 30 consecutive days of mastering the habit of smiling, you will be ready to develop the first of the 3 essential habits of the mind – the habit of mindfulness.

Part II

THREE ESSENTIAL HABITS FOR THE MIND

"The man who acquires the ability to take full possession of his own mind may take possession of anything else to which he is justly entitled."

~ Andrew Carnegie

Mindfulness

THE HABIT OF BEING MINDFUL

"The most precious gift we can offer others is our presence. When mindfulness embraces those we love, they will bloom like flowers."

~ Thich Nhat Hanh

Welcome to the habit of being mindful. The habit of being mindful may be difficult to understand, so I will do my best to maintain a simple writing style. You may need to read this chapter several times in order for you to fully grasp the concepts that are laid forth. Once you do grasp the concepts of mindfulness, I assure you that your life will never be the same. However, just understanding mindfulness is not enough, you will need to apply it in order for it to have a positive impact on your life. Fortunately, you now know of a method (Habit Watch) which you can use to do so easily.

     Even though I have placed mindfulness in part 2, Three Essential Habits for the Mind, it encompasses all three parts of the human being – physical, mental, and spiritual. To become mindful, it is necessary to understand the role of each of these 3 parts. To understand the role of these 3 parts, one should first view them separately and then find the best way to integrate them as a whole. I have used this exact strategy in this book by dividing it into these 3 main parts and at the same time, I show you how they are all integrated.

     In the quote above, the word 'presence' means to be fully present or mindful. When a person becomes mindful, they become like a fully bloomed flower. A fully bloomed human being lives life with all their BEING – body, mind, and spirit. To live in such a manner is powerful, and by living your life powerfully, you show others how to do the same. This is why our presence is the most precious gift we can offer others.

     Within you, you have great power. This power can shape your habits, your character, and ultimately your life. In the Star Wars movie series, Jedi Master Yoda would always preach to his Jedi Knights to remain MINDFUL. He understood that the Jedi would be far more powerful if they did so. Being mindful would help the Jedi to have better control over their mind, body and emotions. And most importantly, being mindful would open the door for the FORCE to flow through them. In this chapter, you will learn many reasons why there is such great power in BEING MINDFUL!

MINDFULNESS

WHAT IS THE HABIT OF BEING MINDFUL?

Mindfulness & Unconsciousness

"A life lived of choice is a life of conscious action. A life lived of chance is a life of unconscious creation."

~ Neale Donald Walsch

  Mindfulness is a state of being where you are highly aware or conscious. As previously mentioned, the purpose of the Habit Watch is to bring you into a state of mindfulness. This is because you are able to make conscious decisions or choices while in a mindful state. A conscious choice is deemed conscious when you are fully present. In other words, a conscious choice is made with your whole being – body, mind, and spirit.

  Unconsciousness is the opposite of mindfulness. In a state of unconsciousness, your thoughts, feelings and actions are on auto pilot. In other words, your choices are of the unconscious kind. Unconscious choices are made without your awareness and thus you do not know WHY you have made them. Unconscious choices are reactive. It is similar to an instinctive reflex. For example, someone says something trivial to you and you explode, answering back with rage and irritation. Once you have calmed down, you might begin to wonder why you had lost control in the first place. And most of the time, you cannot even remember the reason. When you live in this manner, you are allowing yourself to be controlled by circumstance and chance.

  In contrast, conscious choices are proactive. They are made with conscious thought, feeling, and action. You are aware of the choices you make and you know why you make them. In other words, you are in complete control of your choices. And when you are in complete control of your choices, you do not allow circumstance and chance to direct your life.

Mindfulness and Wholeness

To be truly mindful or present, you must be so with all your being – body, mind and spirit. You cannot neglect any one of these parts if you want to lead a rich life. Why? Well, it is similar to having a team of 3 players and only one or two of them play. For obvious reasons, having 3 players are better than only having one or two. If your team is always shorthanded, then your odds of being successful are decreased.

What is even worse is when the 3 players are not playing as a team. When your spirit wants one thing, your mind wants something else, and your body disagrees with them both, you are in a lot of trouble. To be mindful means to be a COACH for this 3 player team. It is your job to ensure all your players are on the same game plan. Fortunately, this book is a manual that shows you how to start doing this effectively.

Mindfulness and Meditation

Meditation is the practice of being mindful. There are various forms of meditation and many reasons to meditate but the main reason, for this chapter, is to learn to quiet the mind. Quieting the mind means to stop the flow of your thoughts. Yes, it is possible to stop thinking, and doing so is the first step in taking control of the mind. For a lot of people, this might be a new concept, but with practice, you will realize that you can detach yourself from your thoughts and quiet your mind.

WHY DEVELOP THE HABIT OF BEING MINDFUL?

Mindfulness and the Ego

"If you do not conquer self, you will be conquered by self."

~ Napoleon Hill

The quote above means that if you (in a mindful state) do not conquer self (you in an unconscious state), then you will be conquered by this unconscious state. Every time you fall into a state of unconsciousness, you risk making choices that may or may not serve you for the better. Mastering the habit of being mindful will eliminate this risk. In truth, mastering the habit of mindfulness is the ultimate way to master or conquer self. What is your unconscious self and why is it such a risk to let it run your life?
The unconscious self has often been referred to as the ego. The ego is made up of your mental programming (accumulation of beliefs, opinions, experiences, etc.) and, therefore, you could be making choices based on an unconscious influence of a parent, friend, teacher, television program, etc. This is problematic because many of these unconscious influences are negative and will serve your life for the worse. The bottom line is, when you live

unconsciously, you are not in control of your choices and you are not in control of your life! If you wish to take control of your life, you must use the Habit Watch to adopt the habit of being mindful.

Essentially, every time you hear the Habit Watch sound, it is a wake up call into a higher state of awareness. The Habit Watch allows you to step outside of yourself and observe what you are currently thinking, feeling or doing. Think of it as getting a bird's eye view of yourself. By doing this, you will begin to realize that you have the ability to control your thoughts, feelings, and actions. This technique gives you extraordinary power - the power to master yourself. And self-mastery is of the upmost importance if you wish to live the life you have always dreamed of or desired.

Mindfulness and Life

"Until you make the unconscious conscious, it will direct your life and you will call it fate."

~ Carl Jung

One of God's greatest gifts to human beings is free will. Free will means having the freedom to choose at will. There are two ways in which you can exercise this freedom to choose – 1) consciously, or 2) unconsciously. Therefore, the first choice you have is – TO BE conscious or NOT TO BE conscious. This primary choice will determine whether you are going to lead your life as a 'Captain' of your ship or as a 'Passenger'.

What exactly is the difference between a Captain and a Passenger? Imagine that your life is represented by a ship at sea. Your ship floats on the water without you having to think about it. If this represents all that life is to you, then you are alive but you are just a Passenger at sea. If instead, you believe life is more than just drifting about aimlessly at sea, then you can become Captain of your ship.

      A Passenger waits for the waves to take them from here to there. They hope that the waves will take them to their desired destination. When they do not end up where they want to be, they blame circumstance and claim bad luck. Thus, Passengers have no control over where they are going, thereby, falling victim to circumstance. Their life becomes one of chance where waves, other ships, rocks and winds all push them to and fro. Where their ship is going or where it will end up nobody knows. This is the meaning of living an unconscious life.

      In contrast, a Captain of a ship will take the helm and steer it toward a destination of their choice. They have control both of their ship and of their destination. Even though a Captain cannot control things like waves, they can effectively cut through them or steer clear of them. And even if a huge storm knocks them off course, they will eventually get back on course toward the destination of their choice. This is the meaning of living a conscious life. A Captain of a ship is the master of their life.

      If you choose to be Captain of your ship, then you will be making many more choices throughout your lifetime. If instead, you choose to be a Passenger, then your choice is always the same, which is to avoid taking responsibility of where your life is going and leave it up to chance. Furthermore, you will let other people dictate your life for you. You will allow circumstances alone to shape your destiny and thus, choice is virtually non-existent. In other words, you choose the life of a victim.

      As for being a Captain, there are many differences

in the way you will lead your life. Once you have taken the helm, you will be making countless choices in three main areas. These are the only three things you have control of in your life. They are your thoughts, feelings and deeds. No one or nothing on earth can tell you what to think. It is your choice to think whatever (and whenever) you desire. The same principles also apply to your feelings and actions.

As for being a Passenger, I hope I can convince you to choose otherwise and be mindful. This is easier to do than you might think. Actually, you have already been using mindfulness by having developed the first 3 habits of this book. Every time you hear the Habit Watch and you observe your posture, breathing and facial expression, you are being mindful. You are being mindful of what you are doing at the moment. And when you consciously choose to change your posture, breathing and facial expression for the better, you are living as the Captain of your ship. You can do it!

Fig. 14

CAPTAIN OR PASSENGER?

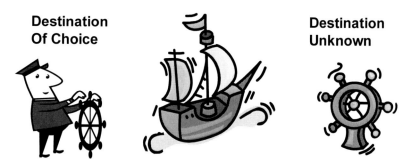

"I can't change the direction of the wind, but I can adjust my sails to always reach my destination."
~ **Jimmy Dean**

MINDFULNESS

Mindfulness and Practicality

When you are in a state of mindfulness, all of your senses are heightened. In other words, your abilities to listen, see, think, smell, taste, move, feel, etc., are enhanced. Each sense is extraordinary in its own way and it is baffling that they are commonly taken for granted. You use these abilities every single day and thus their magnificent value should be self-evident. However, it is usually not evident until one or more of these abilities are either temporarily or permanently lost. For instance, I am sure you have had the experience of eating a delicious meal that you could not enjoy because an illness had numbed your sense of taste. With mindfulness, you learn not to take these abilities for granted and to experience them more fully.

Have you ever tried to listen to a radio station that had a lot of static? The static can cause you to miss portions of the broadcast possibly allowing important information to go unheard or to be misinterpreted, right? In the same way, you may not absorb essential information that is being communicated to you by others because of incessant thoughts running wildly about in your mind. These wild and involuntary thoughts are the static of the mind. Mindfulness may be likened to the antenna of the radio because when it is used properly, it can clear the static of incessant thoughts and the information projected can be clearly heard. With mindfulness, you will be ready to listen without any thought interference which will prove to be advantageous in many areas of your life. Below are some real life examples of how mindfulness can improve your life:

- **Students:** Mindfulness can be used by the student

during a lecture to better absorb important information. It is common for students to become distracted by their thoughts and as a result, they lose focus. You may have heard this referred to as 'daydreaming' which basically means that the student is following the thoughts in their mind instead of the lecture. Daydreaming should be avoided as it can prove to be a very disruptive habit for learning. The Habit Watch will make sure to wake you up from any daydream so that you remain focused on what is important.

- **Athletes:** Athletes should utilize the habit of being mindful if they wish to play at the top of their game. Athletes are constantly using their senses and abilities; therefore, mindfulness can assist them in countless ways. For example, a hockey player must remain mindful of the players on the other team to avoid receiving any devastating body checks while carrying or passing the puck. In addition, mindfulness allows the athlete to remain focused and more prepared for the unexpected. This is also exemplified in martial arts where the unexpected is ever-present, which is why Grand Masters teach their students mindfulness meditation.

- **Salespeople:** Mindfulness can be used to improve communication skills which strengthen the salespersons' salesmanship. A common problem with communication in sales is a lack of presence. To be fully present in a sale means to be mindful of the communication they are sending and receiving. There are many variables in communication to be mindful of, such as emotion, tone of voice, body language and facial expression, etc. These communication variables should be used and observed carefully as even the slightest misuse or misinterpretation of them can result in the loss of a sale. By better understanding what their prospects are communicating, the salesperson's chances of giving (selling) them exactly what they want or need increases considerably.

Mindfulness and Energy

Every thought that is released by your mind uses energy. If you allow your unconscious thoughts to run wild in your mind, they will drain your energy because ceaseless thinking is stressful. Furthermore, the more negative your unconscious thoughts are, the more draining they will be. The subconscious mind records everything you have ever heard in your lifetime. It can play back any one of these recordings in your mind. However, a lot of these unconscious thoughts playing in your mind are not necessarily your own. They could have come from a highly negative influence saying things like "you will never amount to anything in your life", "you will always be a failure", and "you are so stupid", etc. Such thoughts can be very damaging and extremely draining. When you are not mindful, these types of thoughts can roam free, causing major chaos.

When the above thoughts are dominating your mind, what do you think you will attract? Do you think you will be confident in asking someone out on a date? Do you think you will be relaxed during a job interview? Do you think you will enjoy playing a board game that requires intelligence? It is highly unlikely.

ONE HABIT AT A TIME

Your thoughts have the ability to change your mood and your actions. For example, there is someone you enjoy being around and you decide that you wish to ask them out on a date. However, when the time approaches to ask, your mind begins to release some unconscious thoughts like "you are not attractive", "he/she does not like you", and "you are going to embarrass him/her and then your friendship will never be the same again", etc. All of a sudden you begin feeling very nervous. You become so nervous that you do not even end up asking at all. This is how unconscious thoughts can manipulate you.

This time, using the exact same situation, you remain conscious of your thoughts. You do not allow any unconscious thoughts to interfere with your decision. In addition, you use the first 3 habits you have developed and you focus on feeling confident, relaxed and joyful. You approach this person with whom you feel wonderful to be around and ask them out on a date. It is irrelevant whether or not the person accepts your invitation. The important thing is that you did what you wanted and decided to do.

Mindfulness quiets the mind by stopping the flow of negative influences (thoughts, beliefs, etc.) It will shed its light on them and bring them out of the darkness of unconsciousness. Once these hidden thoughts are exposed, they are weakened, making them much easier to rid or replace. In the next chapter, you will learn to replace these negative thoughts with the habit of accurate thinking. Remember, if you continue to stop the flow of unconscious thinking, you will have more energy and more control of your mind.

MINDFULNESS

Mindfulness and Stress

"Life is the performance of function, and the individual really lives only when he performs every function - physical, mental, and spiritual - of which he is capable, without excess in any."

~ **Wallace D. Wattles**

When your body, mind and spirit are not in unison, stress is created within your being. You must be careful neither to neglect nor to excessively focus on any of the three parts. For instance, the body should be provided with an adequate amount of quality food, water, air, sunlight, exercise, rest, sleep, etc. Too little or too much of any of these elements will create stress within your body. And because the body is interconnected with the mind and spirit, these too will be affected by the stress. Therefore, to avoid inner conflict (reduce stress), you must ensure that all three parts are fully incorporated and integrated into your life with mindfulness and balance.

Mindfulness and the Moment

"Seize the time, Meribor - live now! Make now always the most precious time. Now will never come again."

~ **Jean-Luc Picard** (Star Trek: T.N.G. - The Inner Light)

LIVE NOW! The preceding statement is another very important message in this book. Live for the moment. Live in the present. You will see these and similar statements in many spiritual books. In the context of these statements, to live means more than just to be a living organism. To live means to be in a higher state of consciousness, being, or awareness. It is in this state of being where we are most powerful. The main purpose of creating the habit of being mindful is so that you learn to cherish life, moment by moment.

If you live fully in the moment, life will not pass you by so quickly. Far too often, we are so focused on the past or the future that we forget to STOP and smell the roses of the present. We are so caught up with making a living that we forget to live. We forget to tell the people we love how much they mean to us. We forget how precious life is and take it for granted. So please remember to live your life moment to moment and realize how precious every moment in life is to you.

A Summary of the Benefits of Being Mindful

"During meditation your metabolism and your breath rate go down to a level of rest, twice that of deep sleep."

~ Mike Love

Here is a list of some of the benefits of being mindful:

1. Eliminate the risk of unconscious choices; you consciously make choices that shape your habits, character, and destiny

2. You are Captain of your ship or Master of your life; you control your thoughts, feelings, and actions

MINDFULNESS

3. Stopping the flow of ceaseless-unconscious thinking will increase your energy

4. Giving your body, mind and spirit exactly what they need will further decrease stress; you fully integrate and express each one of these 3 parts, therefore; you live a richer life

5. Living in the moment means living with presence and true power

6. And much more; if you want to live a fulfilling life, practice mindfulness daily

HOW TO DEVELOP THE HABIT OF BEING MINDFUL

Mindfulness and Meditation

"- Nature has come to a point where now, unless you take individual responsibility, you cannot grow. More than this nature cannot do. It has done enough. It has given you life, it has given you opportunity; now how to use it, it has left up to you.
Meditation is your freedom...
...the moment you wake up, immediately catch hold of the thread of remaining alert and conscious, because that is the most precious moment to catch the thread of consciousness. Many times in the day you will forget – but the moment you remember, immediately start being alert. Never repent, because that is a sheer wastage of time. Never repent, "My God, I forgot again!"

ONE HABIT AT A TIME

...there is no place for any repentance. Whatever has happened is gone, now there is no need to waste time on it. Catch hold again of the thread of awareness. Slowly, slowly you will be able to be alert the whole day – an undercurrent of awareness in every act, in every movement, in everything that you are doing, or not doing. Something underneath will be continuously flowing. -"

~ Osho

Since meditation is the practice of mindfulness, it is essential that you incorporate meditation into your life on a regular basis. This is easier to do than most people think or realize. You do not have to spend too much time meditating in order for it to be effective. With meditation, it is more about quality than quantity. Actually, all you need is ten to fifteen minutes of quality meditation and it will be enough to have a tremendous impact on your day. Therefore, dedicate a specific time in your day where you can meditate. If you must, wake up ten or fifteen minutes earlier in the morning and meditate at that time. Also, as the quote above states, you can enter into a meditative state at any moment you remember and choose to do so.

There are various forms of meditation that can be utilized to develop the habit of being mindful. The most common and simplest form is the seated meditation. Below are some guidelines for the seated meditation:

- sit in a comfortable, upright position and preferably in a quiet environment

- practice high-quality breathing

- relax your body (muscles)

MINDFULNESS

- wear a smile (enjoy being)

- empty your mind (of thoughts)

- be present or in the moment

- connect to the source of your being (Spirit).
(You will learn about connecting to Spirit in Chapter 7 – Connectedness).

Note: Most of these guidelines pertain to other forms of meditations as well.

Creating the Habit of Being Mindful

"If you are doing mindfulness meditation, you are doing it with your ability to attend to the moment".

~ Daniel Goleman

The moment you wake up in the morning is the best time to become mindful. If you do not remember to do so upon rising, then use something to trigger your memory. For example, by now you have probably built the habit of putting on your Habit Watch in the morning. Therefore, use this action as a reminder to be mindful. You will notice that this technique is quite effective.

We do not all have the ability to attend to the moment all day long. However, the Habit Watch will help us to develop this ability. When the Habit Watch beeps, it is an indication to do what you are currently doing with all your attention. When you do something unconsciously, it is like you are a robot. You are there physically, but your being is just not entirely there. With mindfulness, it is the opposite. You are there with your whole being – body, mind and spirit. And you are becoming more and more mindful with every physical, mental, and spiritual habit you develop in this book.

When the habit watch beeps, the first order of mindfulness is to attend to the moment and to stop the flow of unconscious thoughts (quiet the mind). Next, focus on your senses. In this state of awareness, you will notice that they are all heightened. Here are two examples of situations you might be in:

> a) If the Habit Watch beeps while you are eating dinner, then I want you to be mindful of your eating. How does the food smell? How does the food look? How does the food feel (texture) and how does it make you feel? How does the food taste? What sounds do you notice? How are you chewing your food? Do you feel full? Is the food you are eating good for your body, mind and spirit?

> b) If the Habit Watch beeps and you are in the middle of a conversation, then I want you to be mindful of the conversation. Are you present? Are you listening to what the other person is saying? How do you feel? Are you judging the other person? Are you thinking about what you want to say after they are done? Are you looking at them and their mannerisms to see what they are trying to communicate or do your eyes wander? If you are speaking, what are you saying? Listen to the tone of your voice. Do you believe what you are saying? Are you speaking from your heart?

MINDFULNESS

There are so many more questions you could ask yourself while in the above situations, but I hope you get the idea. The main message here is that you should become more conscious and less robotic. Do not live your life as if you are just going through the motions, but live with your whole being in the moment. With mindfulness, you will notice many things about life that you never did before. It will become a more beautiful place to live in. As a result, you will begin to regain the same veneration for life that you had as a child.

Emotionalize the Habit

"We who lived in concentration camps can remember the men who walked through the huts comforting others, giving away their last piece of bread. They may have been few in number, but they offer sufficient proof that everything can be taken from a man but one thing: the last of the human freedoms -- to choose one's attitude in any given set of circumstances, to choose one's own way."

~ Viktor Frankl

When you are mindful, you are free to consciously choose your thoughts, feelings, and actions in any given situation or circumstance. Mindfulness frees us from the prison of unconsciousness. For this reason, the emotion I want you to feel for the habit of being mindful is freedom. Freedom to choose which way you want to sail your ship. At this point, you have felt a sense of control over your posture, breathing, and facial expression. And now, I want you to have this same sense of control or power over your self and your destiny. Remember, mindfulness is freedom and our freedom is in our choice.

Summary of Creating the Habit of Being Mindful

- Focus on developing the new habit instead of focusing on breaking the old habit

- Remember to be mindful upon rising

- Set the Habit Watch to beep once every 15, 30, or 60 minutes

- When the Habit Watch goes off, check all previously learned habits and attend to the moment

- Dedicate a minimum of 10 – 15 minutes a day for meditation

- Quiet the mind by stopping the flow of unconscious thinking

- Continue doing whatever it is you are doing but do so with your whole being

- Ask yourself questions about the way you are doing what you are doing

- Feel the freedom that comes from being mindful

- To master the habit practice it for at least 30 days

- You have mastered the habit when you catch yourself practicing it at least 80% of the time

MINDFULNESS

CONCLUSION

Going the Extra Mile with the Habit of Being Mindful

Keep in mind that I have only laid out some of the basic concepts and supplementary reading is recommended. There are many resources on mindfulness (awareness) to explore that further explain the intricacies of this topic. Here are just a few of these resources:

- Lao Tzu
- Osho (Bhagwan Shree Rajneesh)
- Rumi (Jalāl ad-Dīn Muḥammad Balkhī)
- Swami Swahananda
- Thich Nhat Hanh

The following are some great resources that teach and integrate the practice of mindfulness meditation with movement. They also teach and integrate body, mind and spirit:

- Alexander Technique
- C.H.E.K. Holistic Lifestyle Coaching
- Feldenkrais Method
- Martial Arts
- Qi Gong
- Tai Chi
- Yoga

For more tools and information on developing the habit of being mindful, please visit: **www.habitwatch.ca**.

ONE HABIT AT A TIME

Carpe Diem!

      Congratulations! You are NOW ready to use the Habit Watch to develop the habit of being mindful. It is time for you to take the helm and be Captain of your ship. It is time for you to wake up from unconsciousness and set yourself free of it for good! It is time for you to be free to choose and create your destiny. And finally, it is time for you to seize the day (carpe diem) and LIVE IN THE MOMENT!

A Poem by Kalidasa:

Listen to the Exhortation of the Dawn!
Look to this Day!
For it is Life, the very Life of Life.
In its brief course lie all the
Verities and Realities of your Existence.
The Bliss of Growth,
The Glory of Action,
The Splendor of Beauty;
For Yesterday is but a Dream,
And To-morrow is only a Vision;
But To-day well lived makes
Every Yesterday a Dream of Happiness,
And every Tomorrow a Vision of Hope.
Look well therefore to this Day!
Such is the Salutation of the Dawn!

MINDFULNESS

Habit 4 – Be mindful of the moment and feel the freedom of consciousness.

After 30 consecutive days of mastering the habit of being mindful, you will be ready to develop the habit of accurate thinking.

5

Think

THE HABIT OF ACCURATE THINKING

"I quiet the wheels of my mind in order that I may present to the subconscious mind my images of thought."

~ Dr. Joseph Murphy

     In the previous chapter, you learned to quiet your mind by ceasing the flow of unconscious thinking. This was a necessary step to be taken before the habit featured in this chapter – the habit of accurate thinking. Having unconscious thoughts continuously running through your mind is likened to a painter having a messy canvas. It would be extremely difficult to paint a masterpiece on a canvas that is already full of paint strokes. With the habit of being mindful, you have learned to wipe your canvas clean of old paint (unconscious thoughts) and now you are ready to paint anything you wish with your fresh paint (conscious or accurate thoughts).

In addition, now that you have chosen to be Captain of your ship, you need to start thinking about where you want to go. The great thing is, as Captain, you can go wherever your heart desires. Therefore, one of the goals in this chapter is for you to discover the desires that lay within your heart. Once you know exactly what they are, you may set sail for your destination. Also, you do not need to worry about getting lost because you will be using the Habit Watch as your compass. Ahoy!

WHAT IS THE HABIT OF ACCURATE THINKING?

Accurate Thinking & Wayward Thinking

"Thought, like all potent weapons, is exceedingly dangerous if mishandled. Clear thinking is therefore desirable not only in order to develop the full potentialities of the mind, but also to avoid disaster."

~ Giles St. Aubyn

Accurate thinking occurs when you are in control of your thoughts and when your thoughts resonate with your Inner Spirit (or core values). Conversely, wayward thinking is when your thoughts are unrestrained, incessant, and negative (go against your Core Being). One of the main goals in this chapter is to become aware of your thoughts (beliefs, mental programs, etc.). Once you have become aware of your thoughts, you will begin to investigate them through conscious questioning. The questioning process will assist you in determining which thoughts serve you and which thoughts do not. After determining the nature of your thoughts, an accurate thinker will pluck out the destructive thoughts and water the constructive ones.

Accurate Thinking and the Subconscious Mind

It is extremely important to understand the way that thoughts and the subconscious mind interact. Whether your thoughts are conscious or unconscious, they are all recorded by your subconscious mind. The subconscious mind is the soil of the mind and your thoughts are the seeds. Each thought that is released, is planted into the subconscious mind. Once a thought is planted, the subconscious mind transforms the thought-seed into its physical manifestation (given that the seed is nourished). Every seed has a unique blueprint that the subconscious mind reads, processes, and then creates. When a farmer plants a tomato seed, a tomato plant will follow. No other plant will come from a tomato seed but a tomato plant, hence, the Universal Law – you reap what you sow.

The same Universal Law applies in the thought realm. Every thought has a certain type of energy within it. Each thought that you release is planted into your subconscious mind and it will eventually manifest. Negative thoughts will manifest as negative results and positive thoughts will manifest as positive results. As you can see, the plant world and the thought world are very similar.

Furthermore, the farmer does not know the exact intricacies and processes of the soil. This is because it is operated by the Infinite Intelligence. The soil and the growth of life are miraculous. Remarkably, however, the soil is ready to be used as the farmer wishes. In other words, it is up to the farmer to choose the seeds that will be planted. The farmer does not need to know the exact workings of the Infinite Intelligence, but only needs to understand the Universal Law – you reap what you sow.

The soil will not prevent any farmer from planting the seeds of their choice. Likewise, the subconscious mind will not prevent you from planting any particular thought. Also, the subconscious mind will not choose to grow only the positive thought-seeds and stunt the growth of the negative thought-seeds. This work is your responsibility! YOU are the farmer of your mind! And when you become a farmer that consciously sows the seeds of your heart's desire, then you become an accurate thinker.

Meditation and Thinking

"Sometimes I think and other times I am."

~ Paul Valéry

It is believed by most people that their mind and their being are the same thing. I can assure you, as many spiritual teachers have often said, this is not so. YOUR MIND IS A TOOL! IT IS NOT WHO YOU ARE! 'I am' is meditation. 'I think' is an action. When you say 'I am', you are declaring your existence or your being. When you say 'I think', you are declaring what you are doing. 'I am' is who you are and 'I think' is not. Remember, you can exist without thinking but you cannot think without existing.

ONE HABIT AT A TIME

WHY DEVELOP THE HABIT OF ACCURATE THINKING?

Accurate Thinking and Life

Good thoughts bear good fruit, bad thoughts bear bad fruit.

~ James Allen

If this is the first time you have ever observed your thoughts, you will be quite surprised. Similar to the example of catching yourself singing songs you do not like, you will catch yourself thinking the most negative of thoughts. This is important because what you think about you bring about in your life. Thinking is an actual form of energy. If you think negatively, you will be expelling this type of negative energy into the Universe. The Universe has laws that are constant such as the 'you reap what you sow' law mentioned earlier. Therefore, when you sow negative thoughts, you will reap negative results. My objective is not to tell you what to think, but to simply ensure that you understand how your mind works and the importance of your thoughts.

Thoughts are very creative. We are creative beings because we can harness any thoughts of our choosing and create what we desire. Before we build anything we must first think of it in our mind. In fact, all that we create for ourselves in life is determined by our thoughts. Jesus said "By their fruits ye shall know them." In other words, you can tell how a person thinks by what they have created in their life (character, relationships, career, habits, etc.). Therefore, if you want a great life, you must have great thoughts.

THINK

Accurate Thinking and Practicality

It is impossible to think of a positive and negative thought at the same time. Therefore, at any given moment, you are either thinking accurately or waywardly. You can only be certain that you are thinking accurately when you are mindful. In other words, when you are mindful, you know exactly what your thoughts are at that moment, allowing you to accurately guide them toward whatever direction you choose. And the more accurate your thoughts are, the more likely you will create that which your heart desires.

With wayward thinking, you can get caught up in a whirlwind of negativity and end up in unfavourable positions. Sometimes, all it takes is one negative thought for this to happen as like thoughts attract like thoughts. It is analogous to a snow ball rolling down a mountain. It begins as a harmless little ball but soon enough it becomes a devastating force. Therefore, you must guard against every negative thought or else your mind will be swarming with them before you know it. If you wish to avoid being a negative force, it is important to think accurately as much as possible and this pertains to all areas of life. Here are some real life examples of how accurate thinking can improve your life:

- **Students:** When a student has an important exam approaching, it would be advantageous to use the habit of accurate thinking in these 2 ways. First, while studying for the exam, it is imperative to think positively about the outcome. You must not conceive the thought of failure at any time as this will zap your motivation and the energy needed to study for those long hours. Secondly, while writing the exam, you must use accurate thinking to stay focused and keep your mind from wandering. Every second in an exam is precious and should not be wasted away with wayward thinking.

- **Athletes:** In sports, accurate thinking is commonly referred to as mental toughness. Mental toughness plays a huge role in sports as it all too often means the difference between winning and losing. The athletes that think 'I can' will usually succeed over the ones that think 'I can't'. Almost all athletes have tremendous physical ability, but this alone seldom wins championships. It is the ability to control the mind that allows the athlete to reign supreme. This is apparent in any sport. The next time you watch sports, look for athletes such as Tiger Woods, Roger Federer, or Sidney Crosby, and you will see what mental toughness is all about.

- **Salespeople:** Thought energy during a sale can be the difference between success and failure. When a salesperson is describing a product/service and they wish to increase their chances of success, they should maintain a positive frame of mind. A salesperson must not allow thoughts such as "This person is not interested", "This product/service is too expensive for this person", or "I hope this person will purchase this product because I desperately need the commission", to enter their mind. Such thoughts will emit a negative energy from your presence and they will decrease your odds of making the sale. Therefore, a salesperson should use accurate thinking and not allow negative thinking to hinder their sales.

THINK

Accurate Thinking and Energy

"Just as your car runs more smoothly and requires less energy to go faster and farther when the wheels are in perfect alignment, you perform better when your thoughts, feelings, emotions, goals, and values are in balance."

~Brian Tracy

Accurate thinking is focused thought. It is focused on creating your heart's desires. When you think of your true heart's desires, this will naturally stir up feelings of excitement and enthusiasm. Just like cheerfulness, enthusiasm has the ability to energize you. Think about how you feel when you are talking about your favourite topic. It feels like you can talk about it forever, right? Similarly, have you noticed the difference between reading a book that you find really interesting versus a book that bores you? You will find that you can hardly put the interesting book down and you might even finish reading the whole thing in just a day or two. As for the second (boring) book, you cannot get passed the first page without yawning 20 times. In the same manner, when your thoughts resonate with your Inner Being, you will be much more energetic and productive.

Accurate Thinking and Stress

"Be mindful of your thoughts Anakin. They'll betray you."

~ Obi-Wan (Star Wars Episode II – Attack of the Clones)

How can your thoughts betray you? Your thoughts

betray you when they do not resonate with your Inner Being. For example, your heart's desire is that you will be a good parent to your children and your current thoughts/beliefs are that you will never be a good parent. This causes inner turmoil or stress. These negative thoughts/beliefs are very creative and if they are not dealt with accordingly, they can create that which you do not desire. In this case, being a stressed out and lousy parent.

      You may think you do not have these negative thoughts, but with the use of the Habit Watch, you will begin to expose and catch them regularly. They are very stealth-like. Negative thoughts wait until you are not mindful to begin their attack on your heart's desires. They affect us all. In fact, several times during the writing of this book, I have caught negative thoughts attempting to discourage me from writing. Thoughts of "you are not a writer/author", "give up, this is too much work and no one is going to read this book anyway", "no one is going to believe what you are writing" and much more. Fortunately, I have been mindful of these thoughts and I did not allow them to sabotage the completion of this book.

      The philosopher William James wrote "The greatest weapon against stress is our ability to choose one thought over another." Sometimes all it takes is one destructive thought that goes unnoticed to completely change your mood from positive to negative. However, when you are mindful of your thoughts, destructive thoughts will not go unnoticed, giving you the opportunity to change them. As soon as you notice yourself thinking destructive thoughts, you can immediately choose to stop and replace these thoughts with constructive ones. This practice will ensure that you maintain a positive mood and thwart the unnecessary stress caused by destructive thoughts.

THINK

Accurate Thinking and the Ego

You have probably heard of the terms ego and Spirit. As previously mentioned, your ego is a collection of memories, programs, habits, beliefs and so on that you have gathered from everyone and everything around you in this lifetime. On the other hand, your Spirit is who you are before this lifetime, during this lifetime and after this lifetime. Quite often you may hear the ego referred to as 'bad' and the Spirit as 'good'. However, this is not entirely true.

The ego is only 'bad' when it is **unhealthy**. This is because an unhealthy ego has negative thought-programs and habits that will lead you away from your heart's desires. For this reason, it is highly unfavourable to have an unhealthy ego dictate your life. However, a **healthy** ego can prove to be very useful and constructive. This is because a healthy ego has thought-programs and habits that match the desires of your Spirit (Core Being) which further improves the likelihood of thinking accurately throughout each day. So remember, you can develop an ego (healthy) that can work harmoniously with your Spirit. Opportunely, you can easily reprogram or change an unhealthy ego into a healthy ego by using the habit of accurate thinking and even more so by using the upcoming habit of conscious unity.

A Summary of the Benefits of Accurate Thinking

Here is a list of benefits for the habit of accurate thinking:

1. Create anything you desire – great relationships, health, wealth, purpose, character, destiny, etc. There is an endless

amount of thoughts you can think of; therefore, there is no limit to what you can create

2. Accurate thinking resonates with your Inner Being which is the source of all your energy; as a result, you will have more energy to create what you desire

3. Accurate thinking seeks out and destroys negative thoughts/beliefs which will reduce stress and decrease the chances of creating negativity within your life

4. You can reprogram an unhealthy ego into a healthy one and further reduce the chances of thinking destructive thoughts

5. And much more; because there is no limit to what you can think and create, there is no limit to the benefits you can bring into your life and experience with the habit of accurate thinking

HOW TO DEVELOP THE HABIT OF ACCURATE THINKING

Know Your Heart's Desires

"Know Thyself"

~ Socrates

In order to build the habit of accurate thinking, you must first KNOW your heart's desires. What are your heart's desires? Only you can truly answer this question because your heart's desires are unique and personal. You must search within your own heart to find out what desires lie inside. Please do not confuse your heart's desires with unhealthy desires of the ego. An authentic heart's desire will resonate with your whole being. In other words, it will serve your body, mind and spirit for the better.

This may seem like an insignificant step, but I assure you that this is one of the most significant steps you can take to enrich your life. A lot of people live out their entire life neglecting their heart's desires. Far too often people choose what they think is best for them based solely on popular opinion. For instance, many people choose their vocation mainly because of money or status. They believe that money or status alone will be enough to fulfill their heart's desires. And time and time again, they end up in a position they really dislike. Remember, neglecting your heart's desires commonly leads to a life of unfulfillment, emptiness, and disappointment. So please do not take this recommendation lightly.

Your heart's desires consist of two main parts – 1) purpose and 2) character. When you know what your heart's desires are, you will be able to determine which thoughts/beliefs serve you and which do not. There are a number of strategies for discovering your desires and I believe writing or journaling, for one, to be extremely effective. If you have never focused on finding the desires that lay in your heart, you may be surprised at how much information will flow out of you when you start journaling. Below are some questions that you can ask yourself for your journaling process, just be sure to answer these questions honestly and wholeheartedly:

1) **Purpose** - What do I want out of life? What are my strongest passions that I would love to live out? What do I

wish to accomplish? What would you attempt to do if you knew you would not fail? What is my destination? What plan(s) will get me to my destination? What legacy do I wish to create and leave behind after I die?

2) **Character** - Who do I wish to be? (Please note that this question does not imply that you should try to be someone else, but be yourself while using the examples of others to guide you in your journey.) What character traits do I admire most and which ones do I wish to adopt for my own character, i.e. Mahatma Gandhi's courage, Jesus' faith, etc.? What core values and ideals are most important to me?

Once you know what you want and who you want to be, you will be ready to determine which thoughts/beliefs should stay and which must go. In fact, any time you come to a fork in the road, you will be able to make those hard decisions more easily. You will simply ask yourself – 'which path leads me toward my heart's desire and which path leads me astray?' The clearer you are about your heart's desires, the easier it will be to choose the correct path. Remember the saying - clarity leads to power!

Accurate Thinking and Responsibility

"With great power there must also come — great responsibility!"

~ **Stan Lee** (creator of Spider-Man)

When you adopt the habit of accurate thinking, you

take on great responsibility. What is your responsibility? To think for yourself; to question everything; to not assume that everything you have been taught in school, at home, or anywhere else is true. In addition, you must challenge your beliefs and see if they serve your Spiritual Essence. As an accurate thinker, you must watch, change and choose your thoughts carefully. This is your responsibility. No one can tell you what to think. An accurate thinker is a free thinker. And remember, a free thinker is powerful beyond measure because they can create anything they can think of or envision. Ralph Waldo Emerson said it brilliantly - *"Beware when the great God lets loose a thinker on this planet."*

Creating the Habit of Accurate Thinking

"As a single footstep will not make a path on the earth, so a single thought will not make a pathway in the mind. To make a deep physical path, we walk again and again. To make a deep mental path, we must think over and over the kind of thoughts we wish to dominate our lives."

~ Henry David Thoreau

When the Habit Watch sounds, it is time to focus on your thoughts. What are you thinking at the present moment? Do not worry if in the beginning you cannot remember what you were just thinking about. The more you do this exercise, the more in tune you will become with your thinking. You will eventually be able to trace back the majority of your thoughts for the past minute, hour, and even day! Thus, the first step is to be able to recall what you were just thinking about at the moment.

ONE HABIT AT A TIME

The next step is to ask yourself, "Do my current thoughts serve me for the better or for worse?" In other words, will your thoughts create what you want or what you do not want? For example, if you wanted to become a firefighter and you caught yourself thinking – "there is no use in trying to become a firefighter because the tests are too difficult and I will fail". Are these thoughts conducive to achieving your goal? Of course not! At this point, do not get upset with your negative thoughts because you are going to replace them with constructive thoughts. Remember, positive thoughts are more powerful than negative thoughts!

Finally, step three is to change the thoughts that do not serve you into thoughts that do. For example, "I will work hard, pass all the tests, and become the best firefighter I know I can be". Now these thoughts are synonymous to what you want. If the thoughts you catch yourself thinking do serve your Inner Spirit, then simply rejoice and continue thinking along those accurate lines. In no time, you will master the habit of accurate thinking and you will be living out your heart's desires.

Accurate Thinking and Influence

AUTO-SUGGESTION

Another great tool that can be constructively used to attain your heart's desires is autosuggestion. Autosuggestion is the process of planting thought-seeds into your subconscious mind. Similar to choice, auto-suggestion is made either consciously or unconsciously. Furthermore, suggestions can come from various sources which can be divided as internal and external. Internal suggestions come from within your own mind and external suggestions come from sources outside of your mind such as a friend, a book, television etc. Whether a suggestion is external or internal is not that significant, but what is imperative, is that autosuggestion is used consciously and constructively.

    To ensure that you are planting constructive seeds, you must remain mindful of your thoughts. When you are mindful of your thoughts, you are able to either plant or discard any suggested thought/belief. For instance, if someone tells you that apples or water are bad for your health, then you can either plant this suggestion or discard it. In the above example, the suggestion came from an outside source, however, you ultimately have the power to do what you wish with either internal or external suggestions - plant them or cast them away. When you know that a certain thought/belief is constructive to attaining your heart's desires, you can reinforce it by repeatedly planting this thought/belief into the subconscious mind. You can use autosuggestion at any time throughout the day, but the best time to impregnate the subconscious mind is at night when you are falling asleep.

    Here are some general examples of conscious auto-suggestion or also known as positive affirmations:

- I am moving toward my heart's desires and I am in the process of attaining them.

- I will succeed in my daily endeavours toward my heart's desires.

- I am intelligent, loving, successful, confident, serene, joyful, and/or any other character trait you wish to adopt.

ONE HABIT AT A TIME

- I will stay true to my core values and live them out each day.

Note: If you wish, you can choose to recite any constructive affirmation when the Habit Watch sounds. When reciting an affirmation, use definite phrases such as 'I am' and 'I will' and try to do so with real conviction. In other words, believe in what you are affirming and recite it with your whole being – body, mind and spirit.

EMPOWERING RELATIONSHIPS:

"Choose to be in close proximity to people who are empowering, who appeal to your sense of connection to intention, who see the greatness in you, who feel connected to God, who live a life that gives evidence that Spirit has found celebration through them."

~ Wayne Dyer

An empowering relationship is one that brings out the best in you. Therefore, it is a great idea to create these types of relationships in your life. However, the foremost relationship to build is the one with your self. Becoming an empowering person yourself, is a prerequisite to forming empowering relationships with others. In order to become an empowering person, you must ensure that you always talk constructively to your self (accurate thinking). Look to your own Inner-Self (heart) for guidance and support. You must become your own best friend.

In other words, YOU must be the biggest influence in your life. No one should supersede you when it comes to making life choices. Only you know, in your heart, what is best for you. And once you determine what is best, you simply convey this to yourself using constructive self-talk. The more constructive your self-talk becomes, the more empowering of a person you will be.

Once you become an empowering person, you will be able to empower others. You will motivate others to bring out their best. What's more, as an empowering individual, you will attract like-minded people and create empowering relationships. These relationships are truly special because everyone in the relationship benefits. Everyone supports each other in living out their passions (heart's desires). Remember, when empowered people form a relationship, the possibilities are endless as to what they can create together.

READING:

"Reading is to the mind what exercise is to the body."

~ Joseph Addison

Reading is a great tool to help you master the habit of accurate thinking. This is because books are a collection of wisdom, experiences and life lessons from people of many generations and backgrounds. There are countless books filled with invaluable information and life altering messages. Furthermore, books have the ability to challenge your current way of thinking or your current beliefs. In truth, you will often come across new suggestions that can improve the health of your mental programming (ego).

The old idiom, *"birds of a feather flock together"*, is important to understand. It signifies that people with the same opinions, beliefs, interests, and so on, usually hang out (flock) together. Another accepted belief is that you are the average of the 5 people you associate with the most! I would consider books (audio, DVDs, etc.) as a part of the five influences because you can hang out with brilliant authors of the past and present simply by reading their material. Personally, I like to hang out with authors such as Wallace Wattles, Napoleon Hill, James Allen, Paul Chek, Bob Proctor, Brian Tracy, Anthony Robbins, Robin Sharma, etc. These are the kind of people I wish to be influenced by the most. They motivate, inspire, and guide people to grow and become successful in all areas of life. Listen to them and they will help you build a healthy ego.

You will find that some books completely resonate with your Core Being while others do not. When you read, be sure to keep an attentive mind. Ensure that you only absorb the information that serves you and leave behind what does not serve you. The quote below gives some good advice on reading:

"Read not to contradict and confute; nor to believe and take for granted;
nor to find talk and discourse; but to weigh and consider.
Some books are to be tasted, others to be swallowed,
and some few to be chewed and digested:
that is, some books are to be read only in parts,
others to be read, but not curiously, and some few
to be read wholly, and with diligence and attention."

~ Francis Bacon

This suggestion does not only apply for books but for all sources of information. For the most part, television news gives a bleak perspective of our world. The vast majority of what is on the news is negative. If I know a person to be negative most of the time, I do my best to change their outlook or avoid them altogether! Since we cannot attempt to change the news' outlook, my suggestion is to avoid it as much as possible. Yes, I am aware that these negative things are occurring around us, but there are also many positive things taking place in our world each day, things that we are not informed about. If you are going to watch the news, keep in mind that, all too often, only one side of the story is being presented.

QUESTION EVERYTHING!

"The high minded man must care more for the truth than for what people think."

~Aristotle

     Only you know your truth. No one can look into your heart and tell you what you desire. Therefore, only you know whether or not an influence serves you. You must learn to assess all the influences that you come across. Do not take anything for granted or at face value. Do not let your guard down. Cast away all the negative influences that have or are attempting to enter your mind.

     I cannot emphasize enough this suggestion of questioning everything as its importance is so immense, it is beyond measure. Do not be surprised when you begin to discover that nearly all of what you have been taught, told or led to believe, etc., is not true. Nicolaus Copernicus questioned the popular opinion/belief in the 1500s that the Earth was at the centre of the Universe, and because he did so, he discovered the truth that it is not at the centre. There are countless more examples I could list where truth is indeed the opposite of popular opinion/belief. Therefore, I will reiterate, do not take anything at face value and always look for the truth through conscious and accurate questioning.

Emotionalize the Habit

"Great spirits have always found violent opposition from mediocre minds. The latter cannot understand it when a man does not thoughtlessly submit to hereditary prejudices but honestly and courageously uses his intelligence and fulfills the duty to express the results of his thoughts in clear form."

~ Albert Einstein

To be a free thinker takes a lot of courage. At times, you may find that you think differently than those around you. This is normal because everyone is different. Just as our faces, bodies and fingerprints are unique, so are our heart's desires. This is a wonderful thing. However, sometimes thinking for yourself can be really difficult because often enough, your thinking or beliefs will be different from those you love. Naturally, this can lead to friction. At this point, you will need strength and courage to stand up for what you believe in. You must not allow other people to forcefully apply their beliefs and ideals upon you.

Parents try to instill their own thoughts, mental programs, and beliefs unto their children. The problem is that what they have engrained in our minds does not always coincide with our heart's desires. Therefore, it is going to take a tremendous amount of courage to let go of any learned thoughts/beliefs that are hindering you from living out your heart's desires. Every time you hear the Habit

THINK

Watch, I want you to feel a sense of courage. You will need courage to travel the road less traveled. You will need courage to create the life you want and to be the person you want to be. And finally, you will need courage to take responsibility for your thoughts, feelings, actions, and creations.

Summary of Creating the Habit of Accurate Thinking

- First and foremost seek and determine your Heart's desires

- Focus on developing the new habit instead of focusing on breaking the old habit

- Set the Habit Watch to beep once every 15, 30, or 60 minutes

- When the Habit Watch goes off, check all previously learned habits and observe your current thoughts

- Determine whether or not your thoughts are constructive to your heart's desire

- Replace any thoughts that are destructive with constructive ones

- Create empowering relationships

- Use auto-suggestion by repeating certain thoughts/beliefs that you know will have a positive impact on attaining your heart's desires

ONE HABIT AT A TIME

- Read material from the wisest people of the past and present

- Always stay on guard and question everything

- Feel a sense of courage as you think for yourself

- To master the habit practice it for at least 30 days

- You have mastered the habit when you catch yourself practicing it at least 80% of the time

CONCLUSION

Going the Extra Mile with the Habit of Accurate Thinking

Recommended Learning Material:

"The Power of Your Subconscious Mind" By Joseph Murphy

P.P.S. Mastery Program – "Find and Live Your Legacy" By Paul Chek

For more tools and information on developing the habit of accurate thinking, please visit: **www.habitwatch.ca**.

Stop and Think!

Congratulations! You are NOW ready to use the

THINK

Habit Watch to develop the habit of accurate thinking. It is time for you to start choosing only the thoughts that serve your being. It is time for you to use accurate thoughts to build your desired character. It is time for you to choose the thoughts that will lead you toward your desired purpose! And finally, it is time for you to have the courage to stop and think for YOURSELF!

Habit 5 – Think accurately and feel a sense of courage while doing so.

After 30 consecutive days of mastering the habit of accurate thinking, you will be ready to develop the habit of affirmative action.

Action

THE HABIT OF AFFIRMATIVE ACTION

"The minute you choose to do what you really want to do it's a different kind of life."

~ R. Buckminster Fuller

At this point, you have become mindful of the moment and your thoughts. Now it is time to become mindful of your actions. With the habit of accurate thinking, you learned to plant the thought-seeds that resonate with your Inner Being into your subconscious mind. However, neglecting the thought-seed will cease the growth of your intended creation. You must learn to nourish and take care of the seed. You must water it with the habit of affirmative action.

The initial step to creation is the thinking stage, however, in order for your thoughts to become a reality,

ACTION

you must follow through with the next stage – taking affirmative action. For example, you may think of your dream house in your mind, but it will not instantaneously appear in front of your eyes. You can envision a detailed blueprint of where everything will be, but it takes action in order for it to be built. This is important to understand because most people will easily complete the first stage but fail to follow through and neglect the second stage. This is the main reason why I promote the Habit Watch Method so strongly. The Habit Watch reminds you to ACT NOW.

In the previous chapter, you were told to find the desires that reside in your heart. This was a necessary step in order to distinguish between accurate and wayward thinking. Now that you are thinking accurately it is time to coordinate your thoughts with your actions. When action follows an accurate thought, you are practicing the habit of affirmative action. And when your accurate thoughts and actions are synchronized, you will become a powerful creator.

WHAT IS THE HABIT OF AFFIRMATIVE ACTION?

Affirmative Action & Inaction

"Iron rusts from disuse; stagnant water loses its purity and in cold weather becomes frozen; even so does inaction sap the vigor of the mind."

~Leonardo da Vinci

There are two types of action. One is affirmative

action and the other is wayward action. Affirmative action is action that is followed by accurate thought. Accurate thinking and affirmative action join together for the purpose of attaining your heart's desires. Action that is not preceded by accurate thinking is usually wayward. It often has no direction or destination. Therefore, you will not know where this form of action will take you.

Action without accurate thought is not always the worst thing you can do. One of the worst things you can do to attain your heart's desires is NOTHING! Inaction is a terrible habit. If you have this habit, YOU WILL NOT attain your heart's desires. Inaction will lead you nowhere.

Please understand that doing nothing is the best option in certain situations. To choose not to act is itself an action. However, what you should avoid is inaction when your accurate thinking informs you to act. For example, you know that exercise is good for your body and reading is good for your mind but you still choose not to do either one. Remember, affirmative action is taking action when your accurate thinking calls for it while inaction is the opposite.

Affirmative Action and Knowledge

"A little knowledge that acts is worth infinitely more than much knowledge that is idle."

~ Kahlil Gibran

There is a saying that knowledge is power. However, this is true only when it is applied or put into action. A lot of people know the importance of maintaining good posture, breathing, smiling etc., but poor

ACTION

posture, low-quality breathing and frowning continue to be the norms in their lives, simply because they are not applying what they know. I distinctly recall, at the end of every GI Joe episode, a character would teach kids a lesson in safety. After the lesson, the GI Joe would say - and now you know and knowing is half the battle. The other half of the battle is the habit of affirmative action – apply what you know!

Affirmative Action and Discipline

"The successful person makes a habit of doing what the failing person doesn't like to do."

~ Thomas Edison

Affirmative action is disciplined action. Being disciplined is DOING what the failing person does not like to do. In truth, discipline is the main difference between the habit of affirmative action and inaction. It is easier to do nothing than to do something. Doing nothing is simply taking the path of least resistance. However, in the long run, you will find that inaction is not as easy as it seems.

The act of exercising greatly exemplifies this point. It is easier to do no exercise than to exercise. Why? That is obvious. Exercise requires energy and work. However, what you focus on or put energy into will expand or develop over time. If you focus on exercising your body today, you will have a better body for the future. In contrast, if you neglect to exercise today, you will have a body that is weak, fat, and more susceptible to pain, injury and disease in the future, at which time you will comprehend the consequences of the seemingly easy habit of inaction. If you are not putting energy into something, it will wither away.

Remember, every time you exercise you are investing in your body and health. It is similar to putting a small amount of money into a savings account. You will not have a large amount of money after a day or a week, but if done so consistently for many years, your future will be richer. This is the 'small daily acts' principle. Small daily acts toward anything can be very powerful. It is the easiest way to maintain your discipline and to create something new and wonderful in your life.

Disciplined action is not short-sighted. When you take affirmative action, you are taking action now because you know that you will benefit from it in the long term. Quite often, you may not like to do the task at hand and this is where you will need discipline to carry you through or learn to suffer the consequences. For instance, you may not like to take out the garbage, but you know you have to or else your house will start to smell. There are always consequences to inaction and, similar to garbage, they usually stink. To have a successful life you need to act now or you will keep facing these negative and often foul consequences.

WHY CREATE THE HABIT OF AFFIRMATIVE ACTION?

Affirmative Action and Your Life

"It is not the critic who counts, not the man who points out how the strong man stumbled, or where the doer of deeds could have done better. The credit belongs to the man who

ACTION

is actually in the arena, whose face is marred by dust and sweat and blood, who strives valiantly, who errs and comes short again and again, who knows the great enthusiasms, the great devotions, and spends himself in a worthy cause, who at best knows achievement and who at the worst if he fails at least fails while daring greatly so that his place shall never be with those cold and timid souls who know neither victory nor defeat."

~ Theodore Roosevelt

Which one are you? Are you going to lead the life of a strong doer or of a timid critic? The strong doer is the one with the habit of affirmative action and the timid critic is the one with the habit of inaction. The strong doer is the individual who has made the choice to become Captain of their ship. They have set sail on a course of their choosing and will strive boldly toward their destination (heart's desires). And the timid critics will watch. Remember, the only way you will attain your heart's desires and the life of your dreams is by affirmative action.

Affirmative Action and Practicality

People with the habit of affirmative action will GREATLY increase their odds of attaining what they desire. Below are some real life examples of how affirmative action can improve your life:

- **Health:** There is no greater habit than the one of affirmative action when it comes to achieving ideal health. You can know a great deal about healthy foods, exercise, lifestyle choices, etc., but until you start applying what you know and making those healthy choices, you will not succeed. It is no coincidence that this book has been created the way it has been. I give you 9 habits that you can use to achieve better health and success in all areas of your life, however, I know that the only way you will succeed is if you apply them. For this reason, I implemented the Habit Watch Method so you could simply apply these or any other habits at any time. Essentially, every time you apply a constructive habit, you are applying the habit of affirmative action and in this case, improving your overall health.

- **Business:** In business, you can use the habit of affirmative action in two ways. First, you can work 'in' your business and that is by providing quality products and impeccable service for your customers. And the second is by working 'on' your business. Successful business owners know they must take advantage of their spare time by working on their business when it is slow and when there is no one to serve or sell to. Instead of waiting for business to come to them, a successful business owner will take affirmative action toward attracting more customers. There are numerous things one can work on to improve their business such as marketing, sales staff, service staff, systemization, etc. The more you use the habit of affirmative action for your business, the greater your chances of success will be.

- **Salespeople:** A great salesperson will not rely solely on the sales that come to them. Instead, a great salesperson will also initiate (act) as many sales as they can. A salesperson with the habit of affirmative action will almost always outsell the salesperson without it. In fact, this habit can make up for a lack of efficiency in selling. Here is a simple calculation to explain this point further.

- If salesperson A attempts 20 sales a day and they have an 80% success or efficiency rate, they will sell 16 items.

- If salesperson B attempts 40 sales and they have a 60% success or efficiency rate, they will sell 24 items.

As a result, salesperson B will sell 8 more units than salesperson A even though they have a 20% lower sales efficiency rate. However, the salesperson who attempts more sales usually becomes more efficient as they will gain more selling experience than salesperson A.

Affirmative Action and Energy

"When you discover your mission, you will feel its demand. It will fill you with enthusiasm and a burning desire to get to work on it."

~ W. Clement Stone

In the previous chapter, I advised you to discover your heart's desires so that you may know whether or not you were thinking accurately. Similarly, by knowing your heart's desires, you will be able to determine whether or not your actions are conducive. Furthermore, knowing your heart's desires is essential because action requires energy and sustained action, requires even more energy. Advantageously, when you truly desire a thing with all your heart, you will have an abundance of energy. In truth, you know you have discovered your mission when you look forward to acting toward it every day.

This is apparent in the artist painting a masterpiece or the conductor conducting an orchestra. In these two examples, the artist and conductor's actions are considered to be more of a passionate expression of soul rather than merely work. Likewise, when you strive toward your heart's desires, the work that is required will not actually feel like work. Instead, it will feel like an enjoyable release of creative energy. And since what you release into the Universe returns to you, you will get more and more creative energy available for your use.

Affirmative Action and Stress

"Our acts make or mar us, -- we are the children of our own deeds."

~ Victor Hugo

Actions may be either constructive or destructive. The summation of our actions determines our character and ultimately, the quality of our life. When you choose to take affirmative action, your life will be enriched. Conversely, wayward action or inaction will lead to a life of unfulfillment, disappointment and regret. These negative feelings are very stressful to your whole being.

On a separate note, it is imperative to understand that a burning desire is a desire which desperately wants, or even needs, to be expressed. When a burning desire is neglected, it will weigh you down and eventually BURN you out. For this reason, heart or soul expression is necessary if you want to avoid stress and maintain a strong vitality. Remember, every time you take affirmative action, it is considered an expression of soul (a natural release of stress).

Affirmative Action and Success

"I prayed for twenty years but received no answer until I prayed with my legs."

~ Frederick Douglass

      Thinking, visualizing, or praying will only get you so far toward attaining the desires of your heart. You also need affirmative action. The Universe will move your desires toward you at the same velocity that you move (act) toward them. Therefore, if you do not act or move toward your desires, you will never attain them. Remember, in order to be successful in attaining your heart's desire, you must act toward them and the Universe will meet you half way.

      The accurate thought-seeds that you have planted will not spring forth until you follow through with action. In other words, you have to nurture each thought-seed with proper farming (action) in order for it to grow and become a plant (reality). For instance, if you want to be a person of good health, you must do as healthy people do. You cannot build a muscular physique by sitting in a chair all day and praying for it to happen. You must make it happen with exercise, diet and other healthy lifestyle choices (actions).

Therefore, if you wish for your heart's desires to come to you, start moving toward them.

The same principle applies with opportunity. You will encounter opportunity far more frequently with the habit of affirmative action than with any other habit. I am reminded of a gentleman who came to work at the fitness facility where I worked. He was a temporary replacement as a maintenance mechanic. However, I had never seen anyone quite like him before. His work ethic was so outstanding that everyone immediately began to notice. In just a few days, he had received a number of job offers from several of the businessmen (members) of the fitness facility. Remember, everyone notices a person of action. Therefore, if you want opportunity, do not sit and wait for it to fall in your lap, but instead, go out and create it with the habit of affirmative action.

A Summary of the Benefits of Affirmative Action

Here is a list of benefits for the habit of affirmative action:

1. Once you have discovered your burning desires, you will notice an abundance of energy while striving to achieve them

2. Acting constructively toward your heart's desires is an expression of your soul which reduces negative stress

3. Affirmative action increases your chances of success in all walks of life and attracts an abundance of opportunity

4. And much more; since everyone's core desires are unique, the benefits are limitless and will vary from person

to person, with that being said, what could be a greater benefit than creating and living out the life of your dreams?

HOW TO CREATE THE HABIT OF AFFIRMATIVE ACTION?

Affirmative Action and Creation

"Whatever your task may be, concentrate your whole mind upon it, throw into it all the energy of which you are capable. The faultless completion of small tasks leads inevitably to larger tasks. See to it that you rise by steady climbing, and you will never fall. And herein lies the secret of true power."

~ James Allen

  The idea to write this book came to me long before I actually wrote it. It was in my mind and in my thoughts for a few years. However, if I had stopped at that point, you would not be reading it right now. If I had waited for it to somehow magically appear, it never would have been created. The onus was solely on me to write this book. I had to unite my idea and thoughts with action. I had to sit down and write. As soon as I began writing, my thoughts and actions became one, and my dream of writing my first book was becoming a reality.
  I have heard a lot of people say that they could never write a book because it is too large of a project for them to take on. But when I ask them if they could write a paragraph, their answer immediately changes. Of course they can write a paragraph. Consider this; it only takes four

or five paragraphs to equal one page, so at an average of one page per day a person can write a 200-300 page book in less than a year. No one writes an entire book all at once and nor did I write this book in a day. It took numerous days of work (action). But as I have stated previously, small daily acts can add up to marvellous creations.

We live in a world today where most people expect instant results or gratification. This is no more obvious than in the health care system. Diseases and ailments that have taken several years to manifest are expected to be healed instantaneously. As a holistic health practitioner, I do not know how many times I have been asked this question – What is the fastest way to lose weight? The last thing most people want to hear is that weight loss is a long term commitment, even though it is the truth.

Therefore, when beginning any new venture, keep in mind the power of small daily acts. Learn to tackle every goal one step at a time. If you use the small daily acts principle, the chances of quitting are lower than trying to do too much all at once. In other words, do not bite off more than you can chew. Remember, any goal that can be achieved in one day of work is usually not as satisfying and valued as a goal achieved after a year (or more) of consistent work.

Fig. 15

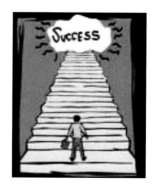

ACTION

The 6 P's Of Action

Below I have listed the 6 **P**'s of action; these are the most important steps to creating your heart's desires:

1) Purpose

"It must be borne in mind that the tragedy of life doesn't lie in not reaching your goal. The tragedy lies in having no goal to reach. It isn't calamity to die with dreams unfulfilled, but it is a calamity to not dream. It is not a disgrace not to reach the stars, but it is a disgrace to have no stars to reach for. Not failure, but low aim is sin."

~ Helmut Schmidt

The preceding quote is one of my favourites. It describes the difference between the habit of affirmative action and inaction. Most people think that failure is failing to reach a goal that they have set for themselves. But here, Mr. Schmidt states that this is not so. Real failure (sin) is having no goals, dreams, or purpose to reach toward. This is simply because when you are reaching for a goal, you are acting and when you have no goals to reach for, you are in a state of inaction. Remember, inaction is true failure.

Step 1 – You must have a purpose to act toward

2) Passion

"The average person puts only 25% of his energy into his work. The world takes off its hat to those who put in more than 50% of their capacity, and stands on its head for those few and far between souls who devote 100%."

~ Andrew Carnegie

It will be extremely difficult to put a lot of energy into your purpose if you are not passionate about it. If you do not have a strong passion for your purpose, the chances of quitting at the onset of obstacles are greatly increased. You must desire your purpose with all of your heart. Your heart is where your passion lies and not in your mind. Just because there is a lot of money to be made in a given venture, do not think that a passion for it will be created if it does not truly lie in your heart. Remember, when you are passionate, creative energy flows through you and into your creation abundantly and effortlessly.

Step 2 – Be passionate about your purpose

3) Plan

"Apathy can only be overcome by enthusiasm, and enthusiasm can only be aroused by two things: First, an ideal which takes the imagination by storm, and second, a definite intelligible plan for carrying that ideal into practice."

~ Arnold Toynbee

Results or change happens when you have a

ACTION

purpose, a plan to achieve your purpose, and finally carrying out that plan with the habit of affirmative action. In the previous chapter, I asked you to discover your heart's desires. Now that you know your heart's desires, I want you to think about what actions you would need to take in order to achieve them. Use the principle of small daily acts. What small act(s), done on a daily basis, would lead to the achievement of your goal(s)?

Step 3 – Create a plan of small daily action(s)

4) Perspiration

"Genius is one percent inspiration and ninety-nine percent perspiration."

~ Thomas A. Edison

Once you have created your plan, begin taking the necessary action immediately. There is no better time to start than NOW! If you do not act, nothing will happen. If you do not move, you will not cross the finish line. To move or act requires energy. It calls for work and perspiration. This is another reason why you must REALLY WANT to achieve your purpose. When you really want to achieve a purpose, you will be filled with so much passion, enthusiasm, and desire that you will have more than enough energy to do the work at hand.

Also, something that must not be overlooked is that too many people wait until they get an inspiration to act. This is a common excuse of inaction that you should avoid. Do not wait to be inspired to act. Inspiration is sporadic and for this reason, it is an unreliable instigator for action. Act now and inspiration will come of your action.

Remember, action generates inspiration more often than inspiration generates action.

Step 4 – Implement your plan of action immediately

5) Persistence or Perseverance

"Nothing in the world can take the place of persistence. Talent will not; nothing is more common than unsuccessful men with talent. Genius will not; unrewarded genius is almost a proverb. Education will not; the world is full of educated derelicts. Persistence and determination are omnipotent. The slogan 'press on' has solved and always will solve the problems of the human race."

~ Calvin Coolidge

There is a great chapter in the book "Think and grow Rich" by Napoleon Hill on persistence. I believe he explains it best. If you have not read this book, I highly recommend you do so. Once you have a goal that you REALLY WANT to reach, then no obstacle will be able to stop your progress. At times, seemingly insurmountable obstacles will come your way. When they do, focus on the finish line and not on the hills you must conquer to get there. When the finish line is the greatest thing in your mind, body and spirit, then the obstacles shrink in comparison and they are ultimately overcome.

Step 5 – Persist toward your heart's desire(s) until they become a reality

ACTION

6) Patience

"Adopt the pace of nature: her secret is patience."

~ Ralph Waldo Emerson

To further strengthen your persistence you will need patience. When a seed is sown, it could take weeks before you even see its initial sprouting. A baby spends approximately 9-10 months in the mother's womb before it is born. Growth takes time, so getting frustrated, annoyed or upset will not speed up the process. You must trust in the laws of the Universe and let nature take its course. First, persistently do the small things you need to do each day and then give your purpose time to grow.

Step 6 – Be patient and let nature takes its course

Affirmative Action and Character

"First say to yourself what you would be; and then do what you have to do."

~ Epictetus

As the quote above states, determine what kind of person you would be at your best and then act in a like manner. If you wish to have confidence in your character, then start acting confidently. If you wish to be a more compassionate person, then start showing compassion more often. Any character trait can be developed by anyone willing to practice it through affirmative action. Aristotle said this a long time ago; *"We become just by performing just action, temperate by performing temperate actions, brave by performing brave action"*

Creating the Habit of Taking Affirmative Action

"And because we are creatures of habit, we must practice. I urge you to practice acting in spite of fear, practice acting in spite of inconvenience, practice acting in spite of discomfort, and practice acting even when you're not in the mood."

~ T. Harv Eker

Set the Habit Watch to go off every 15, 30, or 60 minutes. When the Habit Watch goes off, I want you to ensure that your current actions are in accordance with your accurate thoughts. To be in accordance with your accurate thoughts, your actions must serve your heart's desires. If they do not serve you, then refrain immediately. Begin to act rightly and affirmatively at once. This will move you toward your desires. Remember, by thinking or focusing on your heart's desires, you are giving them power and by acting toward your desires, you are creating them.

What are some examples of affirmative actions? This depends on your heart's desires. You could make a simple chart like the following one for any goal or desire you wish to attain or live out. Ask yourself - what actions lead me toward my heart's desires and what actions (or inactions) lead me away from my desires? By doing this exercise, you will have a better idea of what action(s) would be best to take at the moment the Habit Watch sounds.

ACTION

The chart below gives some examples for two common desires - health and success.

HEART'S DESIRE	AFFIRMATIVE ACTION	INACTION
A) Be healthy and fit	Take the stairs	Take the escalator
	Eat an organic meal	Eat fast-food
	Cook your food	Microwave your food
	Exercise	Watch television
	Walk to the store	Drive to the store
	Meditate	Watch the news
	Periodic stretching	Constant sitting
B) Be rich and successful	Read, study and apply strategies from books on success	Read celebrity gossip
	Create a business (business plan, website, patent etc.)	Wait for opportunity
	Create and follow a budget	Spend beyond your means
	Network	Be anti-social
	Create multiple sources of income	Complain about lack of money
	Set financial goals and create a plan	Live aimlessly
	Organize everything (office, desk, files, etc.)	Let stuff pile up
	Create time saving systems	Complain about lack of time

ONE HABIT AT A TIME

Emotionalize the Habit

"If you can hold it in your mind; you can hold it in your hand"

~ Catherine Ponder

There is always a period of time that needs to pass for thought to become reality. In the mind, a vision of anything can be created instantaneously. In reality, a vision takes time to be created. The single most important feeling to have during this period of manifestation is FAITH. Without faith, a person will most likely fail to persist in acting toward creating their vision. An action taken with faith is much more powerful than an action taken with disbelief or doubt.

Napoleon Hill said "Whatever the mind of man can conceive and believe, it can achieve." In the foregoing quote, the KEY to achieving is in believing. Therefore, in order to achieve your heart's desire, you must have faith - faith in yourself and in the Universal Essence. To have faith in yourself means to trust that you will continue to persist toward your heart's desire with mindfulness, accurate thinking, and affirmative action. To have faith in the Universal Essence is to trust in the laws It has set forth for all of eternity - the main one being that "you reap what you sow".

ACTION

Summary of Creating the Habit of Affirmative Action

- Focus on developing the new habit instead of focusing on breaking the old habit

- Use the 6 **P**'s of affirmative action to create your Heart's desires

- Set the Habit Watch to beep once every 15, 30, or 60 minutes

- When the Habit Watch goes off, check all previously learned habits and observe your current actions

- Determine whether or not your actions are conducive to your heart's desire

- Refrain from doing any actions that are destructive and begin acting constructively

- Ensure that all previously learned habits from this book are being done

- Feel a sense of faith for every affirmative action you commit

- To master the habit practice it for at least 30 days

- You have mastered the habit when you catch yourself practicing it at least 80% of the time

CONCLUSION

Going the Extra Mile with the Habit of Affirmative Action

Below are two of my favourite books (and authors) which have some invaluable information on affirmative action and success:

Think and Grow Rich – By Napoleon Hill

The Science of Getting Rich – By Wallace D. Wattles

Here is an excerpt from *The Science of Getting Rich* that sums up this chapter quite nicely:

> "The essential point to remember is that you must reach what you want by ACTING; by doing things. And today, you can only act where you are, and on the things that are within reach. Do not waste anytime straining after the things that are out of reach, or longing for the things which belong to the future; ACT, today on the people and things within reach today, but act ALWAYS with your mind set on GETTING WHAT YOU WANT. Act in the full faith – the positive knowledge – that you WILL get what you want; make every act a positive act, and an act of faith. Do not sit down and try to ATTRACT the thing you want to you; but begin to move toward the thing you want, and you will find it coming to meet you. Action and reaction are equal; and the person who steadily and purposefully moves forward with one thing in view becomes a center toward which the thing he seeks is drawn with irresistible power…"

ACTION

For more tools and information on developing the habit of affirmative action, please visit: **www.habitwatch.ca**.

Act Now!

  Congratulations! You are NOW ready to use the Habit Watch to develop the habit of affirmative action. It is time for you to start coordinating your accurate thoughts with affirmative action. It is time for you to use affirmative action to build your character and create your purpose. It is time for you to have the FAITH to turn all your dreams and visions into a reality! And finally, it is time for you to start acting NOW!

Habit 6 – Act affirmatively and have faith while doing so.

After 30 consecutive days of mastering the habit of affirmative action, you will be ready to develop the first of the 3 essential habits of the spirit – the habit of conscious unity.

Part III

THREE ESSENTIAL HABITS FOR THE SPIRIT

"If we do not consciously and consistently focus on the spiritual part of ourselves, we will never experience the kind of joy, satisfaction, safety, and connectedness we are all seeking."

~ Susan Jeffers

Connectedness

THE HABIT OF CONSCIOUS UNITY

"Beyond its practical aspects, gardening - be it of the soil or soul - can lead us on a philosophical and spiritual exploration that is nothing less than a journey into the depths of our own sacredness and the sacredness of all beings."

~ Christopher Forrest McDowell

The third part of this book might be difficult for some of you to follow; therefore, I recommend you re-read any section that may remain unclear. The difficulty arises because the spiritual part of our being is invisible, complex and hard to describe in a simplified manner. However, I have done my best to clearly layout the main principles of spirituality. As I have previously mentioned, you must focus on the body, mind and spirit in order to live a rich and full life. To neglect any of these three parts would be unfavourable.

The descriptions that are laid forth on life and spirituality are personal. They may or may not be agreeable with your own beliefs and perceptions. However, I simply ask that you please keep an open mind and really THINK about what I am writing. Take from it what you think will serve you and leave behind what does not. In other words, use the habit of accurate thinking.

In Part I, you learned how to become more conscious of your physical body. In Part II, you learned how to become mindful and take control of your mind. In Part III, you are going to learn how to consciously connect and live with your Spirit. Secondly, you will learn to develop gratefulness. And finally, you will learn how to become a person of service.

Please, do not be concerned about adopting spirituality if you have never done so. Spirituality does not mean meditating on a mountain for the rest of your life. As I have previously stated, I have written this book with the thought of practicality in mind. I will show you simple, practical and realistic ways to be spiritual. I want spirituality to become a regular part of your daily life. And I assure you that this will not be that difficult.

In truth, if you have been developing the previous habits presented in this book, then you are already being spiritual. To be mindful is to be spiritual. To choose your way (thoughts, feelings and actions) is spiritual. Acting with faith and living out your heart's desire is spiritual. Taking responsibility for what you create is spiritual. These were all necessary stepping stones for the habits you are going to develop in Part III.

The quote above states that gardening can lead us to the depths of our sacredness (Spirit). This is true. Once you become a farmer who is in control of your mind, you should naturally discover your Spiritual-self. I will do my best to guide you toward your Spirit. However, no one else but YOU can find it.

WHAT IS THE HABIT OF CONSCIOUS UNITY?

Conscious Unity & Separateness

"The spiritual journey does not consist in arriving at a new destination where a person gains what he did not have, or becomes what he is not. It consists in the dissipation of one's own ignorance concerning one's self and life, and the gradual growth of that understanding which begins the spiritual awakening. The finding of God is a coming to one's self."

~ Aldous Huxley

Conscious unity is the conscious inclusion of your Spirit-self. It is choosing to live with Spirit. This can be done in many ways such as meditation, prayer, and singing. In contrast, separateness is a neglect or avoidance of your Spirit-self. This could be either a conscious or unconscious avoidance. If you are aware of your Spirit-self and you choose to neglect it, then this is considered a conscious avoidance. If instead, you do not know that you have a Spirit-self, then the avoidance is unconscious.

For the most part, I believe that people are aware of their Spirit-self, but they choose to avoid it because they do not fully understand its meaning and importance. I do not blame them. There is so much conflicting information about the Spirit-self which leaves a lot of people confused and unwilling to implement this essential part into their lives. Therefore, the first order of the spiritual life is to clear up any thoughts or ideas that keep you from consciously connecting to your Spirit-self. Once these misleading ideas are positively transformed, you will begin to feel the connection to your Spirit.

Your Spirit-self is perfect. You must understand that your Spirit does not need development. It is your conscious-self that needs development. Your conscious-self needs to fully realize your Spirit-self. Remember, it is the conscious-self that keeps people from consciously connecting to their Spirit-self. The good news is that the Spirit-self is always ready to connect with the conscious-self. This connecting process is called Self-realization which will be fully described in the upcoming sections.

Note: In this book, words such as Spirit, Spirit-self, God, Universal Essence, Source and Force etc., have the same meaning. They are all interchangeable as they are all the same entity.

Conscious Unity and Self-Realization

"Self-realization means that we have been consciously connected with our source of being. Once we have made this connection, then nothing can go wrong…"

~ Swami Paramananda

There are two main parts in the Self-realization process. These two parts are your conscious-self and Spirit-self. Self-realization only occurs when your conscious-self realizes your Spirit-self. As for the Spirit-self, it does not have to realize the conscious-self because it is always aware of it. This concept will be more easily understood when these two parts are described in greater detail.

Fig. 16

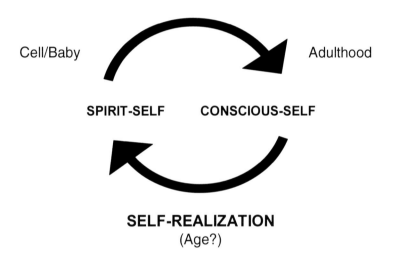

The drawing above (Figure 16) depicts the Self-realization process. As you can see, in the first stages of the human existence (cell, fetus, and baby), you are guided by one thing – Spirit. In these phases of life, your Spirit-self is completely living through you without any interference from your conscious-self (often referred to as ego). There is no interference from your conscious-self because you have not developed one yet. It is intentionally and brilliantly designed this way.

The Spirit-self has an infinite intelligence that human beings need for development and survival during their infant years. If a baby were to develop a conscious-self too early, then several problems would occur. Here are two possible examples of how the conscious-self would interfere with infant development and survival. First, would you consciously choose to breast feed from your mother? In today's society, the conscious-self would find this action repulsive and it would most likely neglect the baby's number one food source for development. Second, would you know how to swim if you were dropped in water? If a baby had a conscious-self, they would most likely drown. The conscious-self needs to be taught how to swim, whereas the Spirit-self knows how to swim for survival.

As a baby grows toward adulthood, it begins to develop a conscious-self. For instance, I eventually learned that my name is Salvatore. I learned that I am a boy. I learned my age and my grade. I was told that I am Catholic and Italian, and so on. All of these things are labels that make up my identity, sense of self or conscious-self.

As this sense of self is created, your Spirit-self slowly begins to relinquish its control over you and your conscious-self starts to run your life. The conscious-self learns from its environment. People, places, and things make up the experiences that will influence and mould the conscious-self. Your conscious-self starts making choices that further shape your character and individuality. In the meantime, the stronger your sense of self becomes, the weaker your sense of Spirit-self becomes. This is because there is so much focus on developing your conscious-self that you naturally forget about your Spirit-self.

This is the stage where most people live out their

entire lives. They live it only with their conscious-self. They have yet to realize that before they developed their conscious-self, they were only a Spirit-self. They have also failed to realize that their conscious-self is something that has sprung out of their Spirit-self. Why is this realization so difficult for so many people?

    The conscious-self thinks that IT is the only thing that exists in your being. Its role is to create a sense of individuality. Self-realization poses a threat to this sense of individuality. Why? The Spirit-self has a different perspective about the Universe than the conscious-self. The conscious-self maintains the perspective that it is separate from all things around it. The Spirit-self knows that this is not entirely true.

    Remember, the Spirit-self is God. Therefore, the Spirit-self is all-knowing. The Spirit-self knows that everyone and everything is ONE. It sees itself (Spirit) in all things. In other words, it knows that your Spirit-self and my Spirit-self is the same entity. This is the spiritual perspective of oneness. (This will be described further in an upcoming section – Conscious Unity and Perception.)

    In order for Self-realization to occur, the following 3 steps have to be taken. First, the conscious-self has to realize that there is another part (Spirit-self) to its existence. Second, the conscious-self must acknowledge that it is weak and incomplete without this other part. And finally, the conscious-self must surrender its sole reign over you and ask to be unified with the Spirit-self. Once the conscious-self takes all these steps, you will have come full circle. You will consciously connect to your Divinity and you will live the rest of your life with Spirit. Amen.

    To conclude this part, you must understand that both parts are a necessity for Self-realization to take place. THERE ARE NO BAD AND GOOD PARTS! Both parts are what make you a human being. Problems only arise when you are out of balance. Therefore, the key is to learn how to HARMONIOUSLY integrate these two parts.

Conscious Unity and Individualism

"You can render to God and Humanity no greater service than to make the most of yourself"

~ Wallace D. Wattles

The conscious-self (ego) has been given a bad reputation. However, you must keep in mind that the development of the conscious-self is a necessary process. The conscious-self is what allows you to make choices. By now, you know that our choices are what shape our individuality. Without the conscious-self and the ability to choose, there would be no sense of individuality. You would feel no need to express your uniqueness.

Please remember that the habit of conscious unity does not imply that you avoid being an individual. Your individuality is very special and it would not have been created if it were not important. To neglect your individuality altogether is to neglect your humanity and this is not beneficial to your being either. In truth, your aim in life should be to express your uniqueness to the fullest and shine as brightly as you can. And you can only do this by incorporating both parts – conscious-self and Spirit-self.

The realization of the Spirit-self does not mean the death of the conscious-self. In fact, it is quite the opposite. The realization of the Spirit-self is the beginning of a new kind of conscious-self. It is the transformation of a human (conscious-self) into a human being (conscious-self +

CONNECTEDNESS

Spirit-self). Conscious unity means bringing the conscious-self and the Spirit-self into communion. In other words, it is a balance of being both human and divine. And what can be better than being human and living divinely?

Conscious Unity and Expression

> *"Most of the shadows of this life are caused by our standing in our own sunshine."*
>
> **~ Ralph Waldo Emerson**

Below are some drawings that describe the human being as a whole. First, I have divided the human being into parts so that I could more easily explain the meaning and function of each. And next, I have integrated all the parts to show how they function together. Keep in mind, the human being is far more intricate than what I have laid forth. However, as you are well aware by now, my goal is to keep it simple so that it may be clearly understood by all. Please take your time and study them thoroughly.

UNIQUE PHYSICAL EXPRESSION

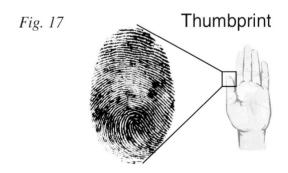

Fig. 17   Thumbprint

ONE HABIT AT A TIME

Figure 17 shows a thumbprint. Many criminals have been caught because they have left this unique piece of evidence behind at crime scenes. Everyone's fingerprints are different because everyone's body or physical expression is unique. Identical twins might have many similarities but there will always be differences between them. The same principle of unique expression applies to your mind and soul.

God has given you a body with certain genetic qualities. These qualities may be either developed for the better or abused for the worse. Therefore, your body will change in appearance based on your life choices. For instance, if you chose to partake in a daily exercise routine for ten years, your body would look very different versus neglecting exercise for 10 years. Therefore, you have been given a unique body that you can further individualize with your daily choices/habits.

UNIQUE MIND EXPRESSION

Fig. 18

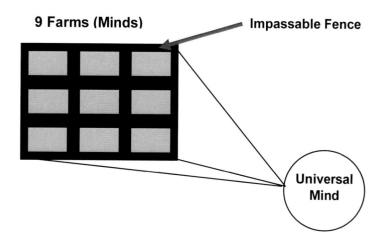

CONNECTEDNESS

The mind is comprised of two main parts - conscious and subconscious. The conscious mind is the farmer whereas the subconscious mind is the soil. As you can see in the drawing above (Figure 18), you have your own farm in your mind. It is similar to having your own body. Provided that you are healthy, you have complete control over your body. You can raise your arm; stand on one leg and so on. In the same way, you can plant and farm any kind of seed you can think of.

The impassable fence around your farm means that you have complete responsibility and control of your farm area. Someone may influence you into planting seeds into your own farm but, in the end, only you can plant them. This might sound confusing but just think of it this way. Someone may only convince you to jump, but no one can actually make you jump. In order for you to jump, you must first choose to jump. Remember, this impassable fence ensures that you always have the ability to choose freely.

The soil is divided by the impassable fence. However, the soil's functions are universal (the same for everyone). If a certain seed (thought, feeling, or deed) is planted in any of the farms, it will react in the same way. Negative seeds bring negative fruits (results) and positive seeds bring positive fruits. Thus, the seeds you plant allow you to shape your farm (mind) which further adds to your unique expression.

ONE HABIT AT A TIME

UNIQUE SOUL EXPRESSION

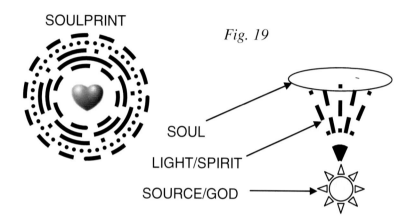

Fig. 19

    The soul is invisible; therefore, this drawing (Figure 19) is just an idea ascertained for explanation. It is at the soul level that individualism is initially created. A soul print is a blueprint for your mind and body. It determines your unique physical, mental, and emotional characteristics. Of course, most of these characteristics can be altered and reshaped at any time, based on your life choices/habits.

    In the center of your soul is your unique heart. Your heart holds your personal desires. For instance, you may really love to sing. Singing lights up your heart and makes you feel great. Therefore, singing would be considered one of your heart's desires.

    Spiralling in and around your heart, you have a unique set of characteristics and talents. Some of the character markings are thicker than others. The thicker the markings, the greater the expression will be. Character markings may be thick for two reasons. Some are inborn while others are developed.

CONNECTEDNESS

An example of an inborn marking is being blessed with a beautiful voice and a natural talent for controlling pitches, tones and notes. These are not to be mistaken with developed characteristics and talents. With enough practice, a person may develop similar talents. However, the thick characteristics and talents of the soul that are inborn are ready to use at anytime. You will sometimes see this in very young children who are already able to sing better than some professionals that have many years of practice and experience.

UNIVERSAL SOURCE OF EXPRESSION

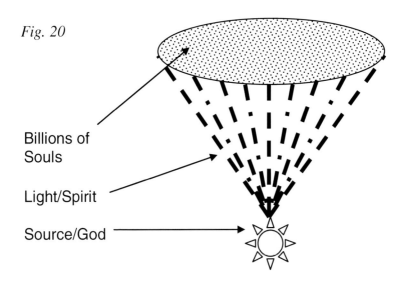

Fig. 20

God is the source of all creation. God is the Light that brings life to the soul so that it may be expressed. Without the Light, there would be no soul or soul expression. The Light allows billions of souls to be expressed simultaneously as shown in figure 20. All of

ONE HABIT AT A TIME

these souls are unique and they have control over their expression.

INTEGRATION OF EXPRESSION

Fig. 21

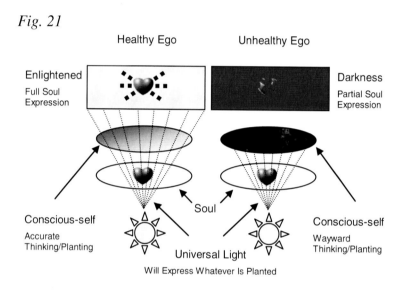

Illustrated above (Figure 21) is the integration of the parts described earlier and the difference between a healthy and unhealthy conscious-self (ego). Life as we know it begins at the Universal Source. The Source shines its Light through your soul and it is then expressed on the screen of life. When the Light is not obstructed and allowed to pass through you, your unique soul expression will be clearly projected onto the screen of life. If instead, the Light is not allowed to pass through you, then your unique soul expression will be dark and unclear. The only thing that blocks the Light is an unhealthy ego.

The ego is shown as a lens that is placed over the soul. After the Light passes through your soul, it then passes through your ego (lens) and onto the screen of life. When your ego (lens) is healthy (clear), the Light will shine through easily and your unique soul is fully expressed. Thoughts, feelings, and deeds that resonate with your heart's desire are what keep your lens clean. In contrast, when the ego is unhealthy (muddied), the Light is partially blocked and your soul is not fully expressed. This is due to the wayward planting of seeds (thoughts, feelings, and actions).

     Every habit in this book was chosen because it helps you to express your soul more fully. Good posture, high-quality breathing, and smiling help you express your soul through your physical body. Mindfulness, accurate thinking and affirmative action help you express your soul by maintaining a healthy conscious-self (clean lens). And finally, conscious unity, giving thanks, and service help you express your soul by consciously integrating the Light (Spirit-self) into your life. Remember, the habit of conscious unity focuses on increasing the amount of Light that passes through your soul and ego (lens) and into your life.

Conscious Unity and Perception

"Everything you see on earth (Universe) is made from one original substance, out of which all things proceed. New forms are constantly being made, and older ones are dissolving, but all are shapes assumed by one thing."

~ Wallace D. Wattles

     To have conscious unity you must learn to see from two perspectives – separateness and oneness. The separateness perspective is derived from the conscious-self. Everyone that develops a conscious-self becomes a separate individual with the ability to think, feel, and act as they choose. This is apparent all around us. For instance, you can walk in one direction and someone else in another. Therefore, anyone who has a sense of self or individuality will naturally have this perspective.

On the other hand, there is the oneness perspective. This perspective holds the idea that everything in the Universe is ONE entity. The oneness perspective is not apparent. This is because the one original substance (Spirit) that permeates all things is invisible. For this reason, a lot of people have a hard time believing and adopting this perspective. However, when you consciously connect to this Spirit substance, you will know that this perspective also exists.

Here is an analogy to explain both the perspective of separation and the perspective of oneness. Two drops of water splash up from the ocean and they see each other. Visually, they are separate from each other. They now have a sense of individuality. However, even though they are currently separate they are both made up of the same substance. They both came from the same place (ocean) and to which they will eventually return. Our human existence is very similar.

Fig. 22

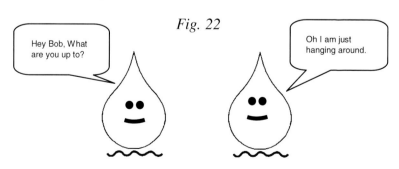

CONNECTEDNESS

WHY DEVELOP THE HABIT OF CONSCIOUS UNITY?

Conscious Unity and Life

"Just as a candle cannot burn without fire, men cannot live without a spiritual life."

~ Buddha

Without the Spirit-self our soul, mind, or body could not be fully expressed. Therefore, you will not know what living truly means until you start to consciously integrate your Spirit-self. As I have often repeated, neglect any part; physical, mental, or spiritual and you will live your life incompletely. When your choices are focused on the development and benefit of all 3 parts, then there will be harmony within. For instance, in one day you may choose to exercise for the body, read for the mind and pray for the spirit. All of these things support you as a whole. Remember, when you learn to harmoniously integrate your body, mind and spirit, you will LIVE a heavenly life.

Conscious Unity and Practicality

Another great aspect of your Spirit-self is that you may call upon it at will. It does not ever get tired of helping you because its energy is boundless. In truth, your Spirit-self loves it when you call upon it. Its eternal light shines brightly so that you may express your soul as much as you wish. If you wish to succeed in any area of life, your Spirit-self will light up the path to get you there.

ONE HABIT AT A TIME

Below are some real life examples of how conscious unity can improve your life:

- **Relationships:** When you are aware that everything in and around you is made up of the same substance, you naturally begin to respect it all. Your relationships will be much deeper than simply the individualized labels you have learned to create for everyone and everything. When you learn to look at each person as a Divine being, interconnected with yourself and the rest of the universe, all adverse judgments will be lessened and love, peace, forgiveness or any other positive feeling will flow out of you with greater ease.

- **Business:** Far too often, people go into business with their body and mind but fail to include their spirit. Once again, body, mind and spirit are necessary in all areas of life in order to become truly successful. The spirit is what drives both the mind and body, therefore, it would be wise to choose to be in business that you passionately believe in with all of your heart. The more strongly your spirit feels about the business, the stronger the drive will be for it to be successfully expressed. When you go into business, remember to consciously connect with God, and you can create anything your heart desires. If God was your business partner, what would you create?

- **Athletes:** All athletes are aware of the phrase "playing with heart". This is because the heart (spirit) is our main source of strength and any athlete who utilizes their heart effectively is always a formidable opponent for the opposition. The importance of this trait is often recognized by coaches as the athlete who plays with the most heart is often rewarded with the rank of Captain. The Captain sets an example for the rest of the team that if followed, will most likely lead them to victory. Remember, the habit of conscious unity is about living your life with heart which is usually the difference between success and failure.

Conscious Unity and Energy

The Spirit-self is the source of all energy. Therefore, the closer you are in conscious union with the Source, the more this abundant energy will freely flow in your being. And this form of energy is natural. It does not have any negative side effects like caffeinated products, drugs, sugar, etc., and it is not a temporary stimulant. Simply connect to your Spirit through conscious being, meditation, tai chi, Qi gong, creative expression, etc. and you can have lasting energy throughout each day.

Conscious Unity and Stress

Since the Spirit-self is an integral part of your being, life can be very stressful without the inclusion of this part. Through my experience as a holistic health practitioner, I have noticed that a lot of people suffer in their life due to a lack of conscious connection to Spirit. Why? Well, with the exclusion of the Spirit-self, one cannot fully express their soul. And because everyone has an innate desire to express themselves, hurtful feelings (emotional pain) such as anger, agitation, and depression, etc., will build up inside them. Naturally, carrying this emotional pain is very stressful.

If emotional pain is not resolved, it will likely manifest into physical pain or disease. This is because emotional pain (dis-ease) causes inflammation within the body. Remember, to be inflamed means to be filled with anger, heat, or uncontrollable emotion. If anger and other harsh emotions are allowed to fester long enough, you will begin to feel the heat (pain) in your body (spine, joints, muscles, and organs, etc.). Fortunately, all of this stressful suffering can be avoided by simply adopting the habit of conscious unity. As previously mentioned, by integrating the Light into your life, you can fully express your soul and live happily.

Conscious Unity and Emptiness

"People spend a lifetime searching for happiness; looking for peace. They chase idle dreams, addictions, religions, even other people, hoping to fill the emptiness that plagues them. The irony is the only place they ever needed to search was within."

~ Ramona L. Anderson

Until your conscious-self finds the Spirit-self, you will continue to feel a void in your life. Your conscious-self (ego) will lead you to many things that will temporarily make you feel as if this emptiness has been filled, but let there be no doubt that you will never fill this insatiable void with outer-worldly things. The void is an inner-world problem (lack of spiritual connection). Once you connect to your Spirit-self, this void will cease forever. When you

CONNECTEDNESS

live with Spirit, all the joy, peace, and love, etc., that you were looking for, will be there with you, always.

Conscious Unity and Abundance

"Abundance is not something we acquire. It is something we tune into."

~ Wayne Dyer

This insatiable void, continuing from the previous section, is ultimately filled by Spirit because the Spirit-self is infinitely abundant. It is abundant in intelligence, imagination, love, peace, joy, and much more. In truth, our Spirit-self is the source of all that is positive or constructive. Therefore, it should only make sense to become in tune with your Spirit. For if you fail to tune in (connect), you will never truly know all these wonderful things (abundance).

Conscious Unity and the Force

"Use the Force, Luke. Let go, Luke. Luke, trust me."

~ Obi-Wan-Kenobi
(Star Wars Episode IV: A New Hope)

What does the phrase "Let go, Luke" mean? Let go of what? Obi-Wan Kenobi is telling Luke to let go of his conscious-self. He wants Luke to use the Force (Spirit-Self). Obi-Wan Kenobi knows that if Luke uses the Force, he would overcome his challenges.

Likewise, you could overcome your challenges more easily if you learn to use your Spirit-self (Force) in conjunction with your conscious-self. Your Spirit-self is that part of you that has infinite intelligence and endless creative possibilities. So why not use it? Remember, as a baby you used your Spirit-self to overcome numerous challenges. How do you think you started walking?

Far too often, we try to solve our problems using ONLY our conscious-self. It is easy to forget that we have this divine part to our being. Once you begin to use this spiritual power (Force) that you are entitled to, there are no limits to what you can create or accomplish. The story of the 4 minute mile is often used to show how human beings can overcome what is deemed to be impossible. A group of scientists had concluded that no human being could ever run a mile in under 4 minutes because it was physically impossible. Their theory held true for many years until it was first achieved in 1954 by Roger Bannister. The scientists failed to include the power of will, heart, and the Force.

I would like to add something else because I know how difficult life can be at times. We have all had those times in our life where everything seems to go wrong and no matter what we do, it just does not get any better. Well, I believe this is life's way of teaching us this important lesson of letting go of our conscious-self and connecting to Spirit. In truth, the main reason things go wrong in our lives is because we ONLY follow our conscious-self and are not using our Spirit-self as a guide. When you feel like you have nowhere or no one else to turn to, you can and should turn to your Spirit. Learn to draw strength from this unlimited Source daily and you can transform every difficult time into one of peace and joy. Remember, have

CONNECTEDNESS

FAITH in the Force, LET GO and TRUST that it will ALWAYS guide you in the right direction.

Conscious Unity and Choice

"Remember this. When people choose to withdraw far from a fire, the fire continues to give warmth, but they grow cold. When people choose to withdraw far from light, the light continues to be bright in itself but they are in darkness. This is also the case when people withdraw from God."

~ Augustine

At this stage, I feel the need to stress something very important. I am not telling you that you must create a conscious relationship with God (Spirit, Universe or whatever you prefer). This is YOUR choice. I am only suggesting that you have a conscious relationship with God because your life will be more rich (joyous, peaceful, healthy, abundant, etc.) if you choose to do so. It is similar to the postural suggestion I made in the first chapter. If you choose upright posture, then your life will be richer (more energy, better breathing, etc.). If you are still sceptical, GREAT! That means you are thinking.

However, please do not just think. ACT! Try these habits out for yourself. There is no greater teacher than EXPERIENCE! I am confident that everyone will have a positive experience with each habit. This is because I have done my best to choose the most beneficial and life-changing habits a person can build. And this habit of becoming consciously connected to and living with Spirit has the power to SIGNIFICANTLY change your life.

Furthermore, I would like to emphasize that God is always ready to connect. Unfortunately, a lot of people have been misguided and have developed a fear of God. Mainly, they are afraid that God has and continues to judge them. Therefore, they feel ashamed, guilty and unwilling to form a relationship with God because they believe that God does not want a relationship with a 'sinner'. In other words, they feel unworthy of God's love. However, this is not an accurate belief. God loves each and every one of us UNCONDITIONALLY and no matter how far you have wandered away from God, you can always draw near the moment you decide to do so. Jesus described this a very long time ago when he said, "Draw nigh to God, and He will draw nigh to you." (James 4:7-8)

Summary of the Benefits of Conscious Unity

1. By integrating the third piece of your being – spirit, your life will be more complete

2. You will have more free flowing energy when you practice conscious unity with the Source of all energy

3. With a strong conscious connection to Spirit, you can fully express your soul and further reduce stress and suffering

4. Fill the emptiness that plagues your heart with Spirit and not with temporary gratifications

5. You will have a more abundant life when you are in tune with the Source of all creation

CONNECTEDNESS

6. Use the Force and you will overcome more challenges than by using the conscious-self alone

7. Choose to live in proximity with Spirit and you will be warm and enlightened; choose to live far from Spirit and you will be cold and in the dark

8. And much more, because Spirit is the source of all that is beneficial, the benefits to adopting the habit of conscious unity are endless

HOW TO DEVELOP THE HABIT OF CONSCIOUS UNITY

Creating the Habit of Conscious Unity

"Resolve that you will now lay aside all else and concentrate upon the attainment of conscious unity with God."

~ Wallace D. Wattles

The first step in developing conscious unity is to decide WHOLEHEARTEDLY (with all your being – body, mind and spirit) that you want to do so. Once you have made the decision to practice conscious unity, you must pledge your commitment to this spiritual connection. You can say something as follows:

God, I now REALIZE that I have not been conscious of our oneness. I ACKNOWLEDGE that without you I am weak and incomplete. I will let go and SURRENDER the control

my conscious-self (ego) has, over to you. I will no longer neglect my spiritual-self and I will begin immediately to form a conscious relationship with you. I will learn to integrate my individuality with my Spirit so that I may live as I was created – a human being. Lord, I have held firmly to the belief that I am an individual living entirely separate to everything around me. I am ready to see beyond that perspective and adopt the spiritual perspective of connectedness.

(It does not have to be these words exactly. I just wanted to offer you an example.)

Renew this connection and commitment every morning:

Good morning Lord, my intention is to live from Spirit. Therefore, help me to remain conscious of our connection throughout the day. I want my Spirit and individuality to harmoniously guide my thoughts, feelings, and actions. I wish that your Light may shine brightly through my soul so that my uniqueness is fully expressed. Also, help me to remember and see you in all things so that I treat everything with love and respect.

Once you have decided to develop the habit of conscious unity, set the Habit Watch to beep every 15, 30, or 60 minutes. Every time the Habit Watch beeps focus on strengthening your connection to Spirit. Also, remember the perspective of connectedness or oneness. Everything around you is Universal Essence and thus is sacred. Treat everything around you as yourself, that is, with love and respect.

CONNECTEDNESS

You can strengthen your connection in many ways:

- You may simply ask your Spirit to be with you

- Maintain a clean ego/lens (avoid negative thoughts, feelings and actions)

- You can envision the Light shining through you more brightly

- You can sing to God (a great example is the song Kum-ba-yah which means "come by here")

- You can pray

- You can have regular conversations with God (as you would with a loving friend)

- Recite a Mantra

- Meditation

- And much more

    Regardless of the method you choose to strengthen the connection, it is important to be mindful while implementing these methods. For instance, it is common for someone to recite a memorized prayer without really being connected to what they are reciting or to whom they are reciting to. Try to avoid this because the main point is to connect.

ONE HABIT AT A TIME

Emotionalize the Habit

"Cultivate peace first in the garden of your heart by removing the weeds of lust, hatred, greed, selfishness, and jealousy. Then only you can manifest it externally. Then only, those who come in contact with you, will be benefited by your vibrations of peace and harmony".

~ Sri Swami Sivananda

With the habit of conscious unity, you know God and thus you know peace. When you connect to God, I want you to focus on feeling peaceful. Peace naturally flows into your life the moment you realize that you are not a disconnected piece of the universe. Peace is wholeness. It is the conscious union of body, mind, and spirit. And finally, peace is living in harmony with everything around you.

Summary of Creating the Habit of Conscious Unity

- Focus on developing the new habit instead of focusing on breaking the old habit

- Pledge to reconnect and build a strong relationship with Spirit

- Decide to connect and live with Spirit every morning

- Set the Habit Watch to beep once every 15, 30, or 60 minutes

- When the Habit Watch goes off, check all previously

CONNECTEDNESS

learned habits and notice the strength of your connection

- Strengthen your connection to Spirit by using methods such as prayer or singing

- Maintain the Spiritual Perspective

- Feel a sense of peace as you connect to the Oneness

- To master the habit practice it for at least 30 days

- You have mastered the habit when you catch yourself practicing it at least 80% of the time

CONCLUSION

Going the Extra Mile with the Habit of Conscious Unity

Recommending Reading: <u>Conversations with God</u> by Neale Donald Walsh

For more tools and information on developing the habit of conscious unity, please visit: **www.habitwatch.ca**.

May the Force be with you!

Congratulations! You are NOW ready to use the Habit Watch to develop the habit of conscious unity. It is time for you to consciously connect to the Source of life. It is time for you to be peaceful as you strengthen your connection with the Universe! And finally, it is time for you to start living with Spirit and experience all the wonders that life has to offer!

Habit 7 – Consciously connect to Spirit and feel a sense of peace while doing so.

After 30 consecutive days of mastering the habit of conscious unity, you will be ready to develop the habit of giving thanks.

Gratefulness

THE HABIT OF GIVING THANKS

"People usually consider walking on water or in thin air a miracle. But I think the real miracle is not to walk either on water or in thin air, but to walk on earth. Every day we are engaged in a miracle which we don't even recognize: a blue sky, white clouds, green leaves, the black, curious eyes of a child – our own two eyes. All is a miracle."

~ Thich Nhat Hanh

All is a miracle indeed. Many people fail to realize that everything about life is a miracle. Everything is so precious. Having a life to live is the greatest gift that the Universal Essence has given us. A lot of us complain about life. It is too this way or too that way. But, compared to what? Think about everything that exists. Do you think you could have created the universe better? Do you think you could have created the galaxies, the solar systems, the stars, the planets, the trees, the animals, the microorganisms, the atoms, or the human being any better than God has?

In the previous chapter, you learned to consciously connect with the Creator of all existence. You practiced seeing with the perspective of oneness. This perspective allows you to see the extraordinary in even the most ordinary of things. And when you realize that everything around you is a miracle, you will naturally feel a sense of gratefulness to be a part of it all. This chapter is about expressing this sense of gratefulness with the habit of giving thanks.

WHAT IS THE HABIT OF GIVING THANKS?

Gratefulness & Ungratefulness

"Gratefulness is the key to a happy life that we hold in our hands, because if we are not grateful, then no matter how much we have we will not be happy -- because we will always want to have something else or something more."

~ Brother David Steindl-Rast

In this book, the habit of giving thanks means being grateful for everything that is given to you, whereas ungratefulness is the habit of taking everything for granted. The habit of giving thanks is about thanking the Universe for all that you have received and continue to receive. It also means thanking others for what they give to you. On the contrary, ungratefulness overlooks all that you have and

GRATEFULNESS

only focuses on what you do not have. It also fails to recognize when something is given to you.

Gratefulness and Desire

"Do not spoil what you have by desiring what you have not; but remember that what you now have was once among the things you only hoped for."

~ Epicurus

It is well known that being wealthy does not necessarily mean happiness. This is mainly because happiness requires the proper balance of desire and gratefulness. When desire becomes too extreme, it turns into greed. Greed is a highly negative emotion that can consume you and your happiness. More often than not, greed leads people to do the most terrible things in order to fulfill its wants. However, no matter what you attain in life, greed can NEVER be satisfied.

I want to make something clear. Gratefulness does not mean that you should not desire new and better things. Desire is necessary for evolution. It is the force that drives you to make the most of yourself. What is important is that you learn how to juggle and balance both gratefulness and desire. In other words, take the time to give thanks for what you already have and feel free to ask for more things to be thankful for. Remember, the habit of giving thanks means to live out your heart's desires while maintaining a grateful heart.

ONE HABIT AT A TIME

WHY DEVELOP THE HABIT OF GIVING THANKS?

Gratefulness and Life

"Feeling grateful to or appreciative of someone or something in your life actually attracts more of the things that you appreciate and value into your life."

~ Christiane Northrup, M.D.

You are made of electro-magnetic energy. You attract the people, things, and circumstances that are most similar to your dominating thoughts, feelings and actions. If you think, feel, and act as if you do not have or are always lacking something, then you will attract more lack. If instead, you think, feel, and act gratefully for all of the great things you have in your life, the more great things you will attract. Therefore, if you want more great things in your life, focus on all the great things you have at the present time and give thanks to the Universe for them.

Gratefulness and Practicality

When you do something kind for someone and you are sincerely thanked for your kindness, how does it make you feel? It makes you feel appreciated, right? Of course it does! Everyone loves to feel appreciated because it is a very positive feeling. In addition, kind acts are often ignored and not acknowledged with thanks. For this reason, the people that do give thanks are usually remembered for their appreciation and are more likely to

GRATEFULNESS

receive more kind acts in the future. Below are some real life examples of how gratefulness can improve your life:

- **Business:** The business person will find that appreciating their employees with the habit of giving thanks is the ultimate motivating weapon in their arsenal. It may take some practice, but if the business person can learn to look for the things they can praise, instead of the things that they can criticize, then they will build an extremely motivated team of employees. Constructive criticism is necessary, but it should never be the main focus. The key is to praise highly and to criticize subtly. The habit of giving thanks will ensure that the business person remembers to praise their employees' work and to find the good even in their mistakes.

- **Relationships:** From now on, give thanks at every opportunity that presents itself. Tell the people in your relationships how much you appreciate having them in your life. Let them know that you are aware and appreciative of all they have done for you over the years (or whatever the duration of the relationship). If you want to build great relationships, I believe that the habit of giving thanks is one of the cornerstones in doing so. All one needs to do is practice this habit for a while and they will soon notice a positive difference in their relationships.

- **Salespeople:** The habit of giving thanks is an imperative trait to have for the successful salesperson. First, sincere thanks must be expressed upon every sale as this leaves the client with a positive feeling upon closing the sale. It ensures that they are not just another number for a given quota. Secondly, sincere appreciation for any referral is extremely necessary as failure to do so will usually result in not receiving any more referrals from this person in the future. People that are appreciated for their kind actions are much more likely to do them again.

Gratefulness and Energy

Gratitude is a positive emotion that can greatly increase your energy. For instance, how do you feel when you get something that you REALLY desire? Think back to a time when you received something that was extraordinary, what did you do upon receiving it? One common reaction is to jump for joy as children do at Christmas time or their birthday parties. Why is it that we feel so ecstatic upon receiving gifts that we desire? Well, just before receiving the gift, it was on our list of the things we do not have and upon receiving the gift, it moved directly onto the list of the things we do have. Therefore, our focus has completely shifted to what we have instead of what we do not have. Similarly, the habit of giving thanks keeps us focused on the 'what we have list', which makes us feel more energetic and ecstatic about life.

Gratefulness and Stress

"Remember that not to be happy is not to be grateful."

~ Elizabeth Carter

GRATEFULNESS

Gratefulness is another state of being that is opposite to the state of being stressed. Stress usually arises from taking what we have for granted and focusing on what we do not have. In other words, focusing on scarcity or lack will increase stress while focusing on abundance will lessen it. When you find yourself in a stressful state of being, allow yourself to alter your focus onto the things you have to be most grateful for and you will begin to notice that it becomes difficult to remain stressed as you do so. When you feel grateful, your mood changes for the better. This is because you are focusing on the blessings in your life. Again, it is your choice which side you wish to focus on – lack or abundance, however if you choose to maintain an abundance perspective, it will be difficult to prevent the things you most desire from coming to you. Practice holding this perspective long enough and you will know that the previous statement is true. Once you realize that you can attract whatever your heart desires, there will be no room left in your being for stress because it will be filled with cheerfulness.

Gratefulness and Conscious Unity

"The more gratefully we fix our minds on the Supreme when good things come to us, the more good things we will receive, and the more rapidly they will come; and the reason simply is that the mental attitude of gratitude draws the mind into closer touch with the source from which the blessings come"

~ Wallace D Wattles

One of the most important elements of maintaining

conscious unity is through thankfulness. A thankful person is in close unity with God. As I mentioned in the previous chapter, if you want to grow spiritually, you must consciously have a relationship with your Spirit. And declaring sincere thanks to the Universal Essence is one of the greatest ways to strengthen this relationship. Remember, when you are consciously connected to your Spirit-self, you are connected to the power that will bring you more of the things to be thankful for.

Gratefulness and Relationships

I touched upon relationships in a previous section but I wish to expand a little further here. Sadly, far too often, we forget to express our appreciation for our loved ones. Not just for what they do for us, but also for whom they are and what they mean to us. What if one of your loved ones were to die tomorrow, what would you say to them? Why wait? Why not tell them NOW how you feel about them? How do you think your relationship will change if you expressed your gratitude for having their special presence in your life? As far as I am concerned, I can promise you that your relationships will rise up to a new level. Try it and see.

Summary of the Benefits of Giving Thanks

1. Attract more of the people and things that you desire into your life

2. Feel more energetic and ecstatic about life when focusing on your 'what I have list'

GRATEFULNESS

3. Focusing on abundance instead of scarcity will reduce the amount of stress you have in your life; gratefulness and knowing that you will continue to receive that which you desire makes it easier to maintain a cheerful mood

4. Gratefulness further strengthens your conscious relationship with your Spirit-self

5. Expressing your gratitude and love for others, will take your relationships upward to a new level

6. And much more, the benefits you can receive with the attitude of gratitude are infinite

HOW TO DEVELOP THE HABIT OF GIVING THANKS

Gratefulness and Faith

"Be as thankful for it all the time as you expect to be when it has taken form. The person who can sincerely thank God for the things which as yet he owns only in imagination has real faith."

~ Wallace D. Wattles

A major part of faith is to be able to see through appearances. So far I have been telling you to be thankful for what you have. In the quote above, Wattles takes it one step further and states that if you want something ask God and be thankful for it before you actually receive it. In other words, thank the Universal Essence for giving you what you have asked for as if it has already been given to you. Now that is FAITH!

In the previous chapter, you learned about the spiritual perspective. Everything looks and seems to be separate and independent of each other. Thus, it takes tremendous faith to maintain the spiritual perspective and to see God in everything. It takes faith because you believe in something beyond what appears to be. You believe in unity even though the appearance of separateness is around you.

Likewise, it also takes faith to be thankful for what you do not receive. For example, you are in a rush to get to work and you are catching all the red lights. This starts to irritate you. It appears as if everything is not going your way. However, what if all those red lights allowed you to arrive to your destination safely. It might have been that if one of those lights were green, you would have been involved in a terrible accident.

One of the ultimate calls of faith comes from the appearance of death. The heart stops beating. The breath stops. And the body is lifeless. To have faith means to believe that there is life after death. Just as I had mentioned in the example of the two drops of water, the immortal spirit lives on and has only departed from its temporary home in the body. For this reason, I believe when someone we love passes away, we should be grateful for the time we did get to share with them, no matter how long (or short).

GRATEFULNESS

Creating the Habit of Giving Thanks

"To educate yourself for the feeling of gratitude means to take nothing for granted, but to always seek out and value the kind that will stand behind the action. Nothing that is done for you is a matter of course. Everything originates in a will for the good, which is directed at you. Train yourself never to put off the word or action for the expression of gratitude."

~ Albert Schweitzer

  A great exercise to do is to sit down and create a list of all the things you have and are grateful for in your life. You will be surprised at how long this list can get if you really examine each area of your life. Doing this exercise will assist you when the Habit Watch beeps. You will have lots of things to choose from to thank God for. You will find that you will be able to add more and more to this list as you develop the habit of giving thanks. This is because you will notice things that you already have and are taking for granted, and you will begin to attract more things into your life as a result of using the habit of giving thanks.

  Also, feel free to give thanks for whatever comes to mind or feels right at the moment. Do not worry if it gets repetitive. This is natural and is bound to happen often. The key is to be mindful and sincere in your thanksgiving. In other words, give thanks from the depths of your heart. Below is a basic guide for creating a gratitude list:

CREATE A GRATITUDE LIST

- People: What people are you thankful for being in your life? (i.e. father, mother, siblings, friends, spouse, children, etc.)

- Things: What things are you grateful for being in your life? (i.e. house, money, career or legacy, etc.)

- Life: What are you grateful for most about life? (i.e. the experience, your Spirit, Body and Mind, etc.)

PRAYER

"A simple grateful thought toward heaven is the most perfect prayer."

~ Gotthold Ephraim Lessing

Once you have a gratitude list, you can choose one thing from that list and expand on it using prayer. Again, this will strengthen your connection and relationship with the Universal Essence.

Here are some examples:

Lord, thank you for the body you have given me. I love the way I am able to see with my eyes…or feel with my hands…or run really fast.

Universe, thank you for the mind you have given me. I love the way I am able to remember cherished moments…or think freely…or visualize anything I want.

God, thank you for the relationship I have with my Father. I love the way his face lights up when he sees me…or how

GRATEFULNESS

he has worked so hard to raise our family…or for teaching me great parenting skills.

DAILY MORNING THANKS

"When you arise in the morning, think of what a precious privilege it is to be alive - to breathe, to think, to enjoy, to love."

~ Marcus Aurelius

    A great way to begin your day is to give thanks to the Universe for your life. Usually, I consciously connect with the Universal Creator first and then I give thanks for my life. Once you truly grasp the magnitude of the gift of life, you will know in your heart, that it is right to give thanks and praise. Without a life, you could not be grateful for anything. Therefore, the giving of thanks for your life should always precede everything else. I then give thanks for the blessings in my life that are most important to me. It can be people, health, relationship(s), joy, career, home, love, etc. In essence, I focus on the kinds of people and things I love having, and want more of, in my life.

A Helpful Perspective

    The perspective that I believe supports this habit most is the "Perfect Perspective". This perspective maintains the idea that your life is perfect from beginning to end (birth to death). And nothing can change that. The fact that you are here, experiencing this life is indeed perfect and everything else is just a bonus. Allow me to explain this further.

ONE HABIT AT A TIME

If you write a test and you get 10/10, you have achieved a perfect score. If there is a bonus question and you get it wrong you still have a perfect score. It does not diminish your perfection. In the same way, if you answer the bonus question correctly, you will just be adding to your perfection. Therefore, the key is to always see your life as perfect. With this perspective, you will remain grateful when things go wrong and you will look at things that go right as a bonus.

Emotionalize the Habit

GRATITUDE (Before)

"Gratitude is the inward feeling of kindness received. Thankfulness is the natural impulse to express that feeling. Thanksgiving is the following of that impulse."

~ Henry Van Dyke

In order to have the full power of the habit of giving thanks, you must emotionally charge it with a sincere feeling of gratitude. To give thanks without a genuine feeling of gratitude is inauthentic and weak. Remember, the giving of thanks is a result of the feeling of gratitude. Therefore, the feeling of gratitude always precedes the thanksgiving. For this habit only, I have included an additional supporting emotion. Now that you know how to feel before you give thanks, I will present you with a great emotion to feel after you give thanks.

GRATEFULNESS

ABUNDANCE (After)

"You simply will not be the same person two months from now after consciously giving thanks each day for the abundance that exists in your life. And you will have set in motion an ancient spiritual law: the more you have and are grateful for, the more will be given you."

~ Sarah Ban Breathnach

After you give thanks, I want you to feel a sense of abundance. This feeling of abundance will attract more of the things that you will be grateful for. This is because the feeling of abundance is highly positive and creative. Remember, the Universe is abundant for everyone. It does not favour one person over another. For this reason, there is no need to hoard, manipulate, and/or steal from others to receive. As a matter of fact, those are the traits that distance you from authentic abundance. Therefore, instead of feeling jealous when others receive, as a lot of people do, feel the abundance that is around for all of us.

Summary of Creating the Habit of Giving Thanks

- Focus on developing the new habit instead of focusing on breaking the old habit

- Create a gratitude list of all the things you are grateful for in your life

- Give thanks to God for your life every morning

- Set the Habit Watch to beep once every 15, 30, or 60

ONE HABIT AT A TIME

minutes

- When the Habit Watch goes off, check all previously learned habits and then give thanks to the Universe for anything that comes to mind or feels right at the moment

- Reinforce your unique relationship with God using prayers of gratitude

- Use the "perfect perspective"

- Feel a sense of gratitude before you give thanks to the Universal Essence and a sense of abundance after the thanksgiving

- To master the habit practice it for at least 30 days

- You have mastered the habit when you catch yourself practicing it at least 80% of the time

CONCLUSION

It is Right to Give Thanks and Praise!

Congratulations! You are NOW ready to use the Habit Watch to develop the habit of giving thanks. It is time for you to give thanks to the Source for giving you this perfect life. It is time for you to express your gratefulness for all that you have received and will receive in your life. And finally, it is time for you to feel and claim the abundance that is rightfully yours!

GRATEFULNESS

Be Thankful

Be thankful that you don't already have everything you desire,
If you did, what would there be to look forward to?

Be thankful when you don't know something,
For it gives you the opportunity to learn.

Be thankful for the difficult times.
During those times you grow.

Be thankful for your limitations,
Because they give you opportunities for improvement.

Be thankful for each new challenge,
Because it will build your strength and character.

Be thankful for your mistakes,
They will teach you valuable lessons.

Be thankful when you're tired and weary,
Because it means you've made a difference.

It is easy to be thankful for the good things.
A life of rich fulfillment comes to those who are
also thankful for the setbacks.

GRATITUDE can turn a negative into a positive.
Find a way to be thankful for your troubles
and they can become your blessings.

~ Author Unknown ~

Habit 8 – Express your gratitude by giving thanks.

After 30 consecutive days of mastering the habit of giving thanks, you will be ready to develop the habit of service.

9

Golden Rule

THE HABIT OF SERVICE

"We cannot live for ourselves alone. Our lives are connected by a thousand invisible threads, and along these sympathetic fibers, our actions run as causes and return to us as results."

~ Herman Melville

In this chapter, you will learn another fundamental way in which to be more spiritual – the habit of service. The habit of service is guaranteed to strengthen your connection to Spirit. Remember, the greatest service you can do for others and God is to follow your heart's desire and make the most of yourself. However, it would be unwise to go about this alone. You will find that you are going to need the help of others to be successful. In a like manner, you will be called upon for assistance to help others become successful. And the habit of service is about helping others.

Life is not ONLY about you and your purpose. Your purpose is and should be very important to you. However, helping others find and reach their own heart's desire is also important. Remember, it will be much easier for you to reach your own heart's desire with the aid of other people and when you help others, they will help you in return. People helping each other to succeed – now that is spiritual!

The habit of service is closely tied to the Golden Rule - treat your neighbour as you would want to be treated. To always treat everyone with respect, kindness, and love is not an easy task. For most people, this habit will be the most difficult to develop. It takes a lot of character to follow this rule diligently. However, I believe this habit will be much easier to develop now that you have mastered the previous habits in this book. This is my belief because these habits have strengthened your character and better prepared you to tackle this feat.

Once again, throughout the writing of this book, I have assumed that the reader will choose to apply the habits I have suggested. However, I cannot force anyone to follow the Golden Rule and apply the habit of service. I can only highly recommend it. Remember, the human soul shines brighter when following the Golden Rule. That is why it is called the 'Golden' Rule.

GOLDEN RULE

WHAT IS THE HABIT OF SERVICE?

Service & Selfishness

> *"As far as service goes, it can take the form of a million things. To do service, you don't have to be a doctor working in the slums for free, or become a social worker. Your position in life and what you do doesn't matter as much as how you do what you do."*
>
> **~ Elisabeth Kubler-Ross**

In this book, service means thinking, feeling, and acting, in a helpful manner, for others. Selfishness is the opposite – all thoughts, feelings, and actions are done SOLELY for personal gain and often at the expense of others. The habit of service is simply the giving of something to others. It may be in the form of a blessing, a loving thought, an act of random kindness and so on. The possibilities of service are endless. And the beauty of service is that anyone can do it. Martin Luther King Jr. said *"Everybody can be great because anybody can serve. You don't have to have a college degree to serve. You don't have to make your subject and verb agree to serve. You only need a heart full of grace. A soul generated by love."*

Service and the Golden Rule

The habit of service wonderfully interconnects with the Golden Rule. The Golden Rule is fully explained below by an excerpt taken from Napoleon Hill's Laws of Success book. I have personally framed this Code of

Ethics page and it now hangs on a wall at home. They have become my 12 commandments. I am committed to live by these commandments to the best of my ability. I hope you adopt them too.

Take a look at number X of the Code of Ethics and read it now please. This is what the habit of service is all about! Service is about ACTIVELY APPLYING the Golden Rule. It is being an initiator. It is helping others even if they have never done anything for you in the past. If everyone waited to be helped before they helped others, then no one would ever help each other! And what a frightening world that would be.

MY CODE OF ETHICS

I. **I believe in the Golden Rule as the basis of all human conduct; therefore, I will never do to another person that which I would not be willing for that person to do to me if our positions were reversed.**

II. **I will be honest, even to the slightest detail, in all my transactions with others, not alone because of my desire to be fair with them, but because of my desire to impress the idea of honesty on my own subconscious mind, thereby weaving this essential quality into my own character.**

III. **I will forgive those who are unjust toward me, with no thought as to whether they deserve it or not, because I understand the law in which forgiveness of others strengthens my own character and wipes out the**

effects of my own transgressions, in my subconscious mind.

IV. I will be just, generous and fair with others always, even though I know that these acts will go unnoticed and unrecorded, in the ordinary terms of reward, because I understand and intend to apply the law through the aid of which one's own character is but the sum total of one's own *acts* and *deeds*.

V. Whatever time I may have to devote to the discovery and exposure of the weaknesses and faults of others I will devote, more profitably, to the discovery and *correction* of my own.

VI. I will slander no person, no matter how much I may believe another person may deserve it, because I wish to plant no destructive suggestions in my own subconscious mind.

VII. I recognize the power of Thought as being an inlet leading into my brain from the universal ocean of life; therefore, I will set no destructive thoughts afloat upon that ocean lest they pollute the minds of others.

VIII. I will conquer the common human tendency toward hatred, and envy, and selfishness, and jealousy, and malice, and pessimism, and doubt, and fear; for I believe these to be the seed from which the world harvests most of its troubles.

IX. When my mind is not occupied with thoughts that tend toward the attainment of my *definite chief aim* in life, I will voluntarily keep it filled with thoughts of courage, and self-confidence, and goodwill toward others, and faith, and kindness, and loyalty, and love for truth, and justice, for I believe these to be the seed from which the world reaps its harvest of progressive growth.

X. I understand that a mere passive belief in the soundness of the Golden Rule philosophy is of no value whatsoever, either to myself or to others; therefore, I will *actively* put into operation this universal rule for good in all my transactions with others.

XI. I understand the law through the operation of which my own character is developed from my own *acts* and *thoughts*; therefore, I will guard with care all that goes into its development.

XII. Realizing that enduring happiness comes only through helping others find it; that no act of kindness is without its reward, even though it may never be directly repaid, I will do my best to assist others when and where the opportunity appears.

- Napoleon Hill, 1916

GOLDEN RULE

WHY DEVELOP THE HABIT OF SERVICE?

Service and Life

"Understand this law and you will then know, beyond room for the slightest doubt, that you are constantly punishing yourself for every wrong you commit and rewarding yourself for every act of constructive conduct in which you indulge."

~ Napoleon Hill

Once again, I will shift focus to the dominating law of the Universe – you reap what you sow. When you use the habit of service, you sow seeds of love, kindness, joy, etc., and you will reap like benefits. For example, the person who says hi, on a daily basis, to all their fellow employees will get more employees saying hi in return as compared to the person who never says hi to anyone. We can see the 'you reap what you sow' law all around us. If people are loved, it is because they give love. If people have a lot of honest, reliable, and trustworthy friends, it is because they SHARE these same qualities.

This book is about changing your life for the better and if you practice the habit of service, I assure you it will happen. The reason I am so certain is because of the 'you reap what you sow' law. One cannot sow goodness and reap evil just as one could not sow apple seeds and grow a pine tree. Therefore, YOU ARE RESPONSIBLE for what you sow and reap. Remember, having the habit of service ensures that you will sow and reap more goodness (positivity) in your life.

ONE HABIT AT A TIME

Service and Practicality

In the previous chapters, I offered some practical examples of how each habit can improve your life. However, I am not going to do this for this particular habit because the focus here is not intended to be on you. Of course, there are countless ways in which the habit of service can improve your business, salesmanship, etc., but that should not be the main purpose of adopting this habit. The main purpose of this habit is about serving others to improve or benefit their lives. Anything you receive in return should only be viewed as a bonus and not as an expectation or reward. In other words, when you serve others, do not do it so that you may receive something in return at some future time, but serve because you enjoy helping others.

Service and Energy

"In nothing do men more nearly approach the gods than in doing good to their fellow men."

~ Cicero

The Universal Essence has given and continues to give us life in an infinite amount of ways, i.e. the sun, oxygen, water, etc., and yet it asks for nothing from us in return. This is the ultimate example of service. When we serve selflessly from our heart, we emulate the Divine and we strengthen our connection to Spirit or in other words, we "more nearly approach the gods". And because service draws us closer to our divinity, we will naturally experience an increase of spiritual energy flowing through us. As a result of this increased flow of energy, we will be able to live more fully and serve more often.

Service and Stress

"Be unselfish. That is the first and final commandment for those who would be useful and happy in their usefulness. If you think of yourself only, you cannot develop because you are choking the source of development, which is spiritual expansion through thought for others."

~ Charles W. Eliot

As mentioned in chapter 7, the Spirit-self has the oneness perspective which coincides with unity and service. Selfishness inevitably leads to stress because the Spirit-self is naturally inclined to serve. When you make choices that distance you from your Spirit-self, you will eventually feel the stress of the consequences. Remember, neglecting necessities of the spirit is no different than neglecting the necessities of your body or mind. If you wish to reduce negative stress in your life, ensure to maintain a strong spiritual connection by adopting the habit of service.

Service and Character

"The highest of distinctions is service to others."

~ King George VI

When I find myself struggling with something or in

need of help, I know the people who I can rely on and the ones I cannot. We always remember the people who are there for us in times of need. They are people of service. Imagine how much you would accomplish having many people of service around you. Well, in order to have many people of service around you, you must become a person of service yourself. Advantageously, when you have the habit of service in your character, you will never be short of a helping hand.

Please take a look at number IV of the Code of Ethics and read it. A lot of people will not serve others because they are sceptical of the others serving them in return. However, as I have indicated previously the 'you reap what you sow' law ensures that if you serve a person and they do not directly serve you in return, you will still reap what you have sown through other channels. For instance, a friend named Albertino is moving to Italy for the rest of his life and he asks for my help. If I help Albertino move, chances are, I will never see him again and he will not be able to ever return the favour. But even though Albertino will never serve me in return, I nonetheless have done three things.

First, I have weaved the trait of service into my own character. By weaving the trait of service into my own character, I use the law of attraction to attract others with this same character trait into my life. Second, I have planted a seed of service. This seed will grow and I will reap service in return. So when the time comes that I am in need of service, although Albertino is in Italy, I will reap the help of Charlie, another friend of mine. Third, I have set an example of service to Albertino, who may very well forward that spirit of service onto someone else.

It is important to not have tunnel vision. Always know that what you sow, you will reap. Whether it is constructive or destructive, what you send out will come back to you. It is an inescapable law. Below is a quote that beautifully describes what I am saying:

Talk not of wasted affection, affection never was wasted, if it enrich not the heart of another, its waters returning back to their springs, like the rain shall fill them full of refreshment; that which the fountain sends forth returns again to the fountain.

~ Henry Wadsworth Longfellow (1807 - 1882)

Service and Cheerfulness

"The best way to cheer yourself up is to try to cheer somebody else up".

~ Mark Twain

     If someone were to go out of their way and do something great for you unexpectedly, how would that make you feel? I will never forget the day my wife threw a surprise 30th birthday party for me. I never expected it. I thought it was going to be just another ordinary evening when I walked into my house. Instead, I was joyfully greeted by the people I care about most. Needless to say, I felt ecstatic that day and I still do whenever I think about it. I will remember that act of service for the rest of my life because of the sentimental value it holds in my heart. I am forever grateful to my wife for that day.

     It does not have to be a huge act of service to cheer someone up and make their day. Sometimes a simple hello, a genuine compliment, or making them laugh will suffice.

Why is this so? Well, that person could be having a terrible day and you might be the only positive thing they have come across all day. Sometimes the small things in life are sweeter than the large. Therefore, it is difficult to measure the size of a service.

Everyone loves love. We all want to feel loved. When we serve someone, it shows that we care about them. Therefore, it is usually not the service itself that cheers people up, but the message of love underneath it that does. And when the person receiving the service feels cheerful, we cannot help but feel the same. This is because their cheerful reaction signifies that they have accepted our service (love) and love us in return.

Service and Relationship

In order to achieve great success, you will need the help of others. Furthermore, what is so great about success if you have no one to share it with when you attain it? Remember, part of being truly successful is having great relationships in your life. And service is the main ingredient for creating strong relationships. If you wish to create powerful relationships, you must learn to implement this essential quality regularly. In a powerful relationship, you enjoy helping your counter-part and your counter-part enjoys helping you. In addition, both parties help to bring out the best in each other and this leads to a higher quality of life for everyone involved.

GOLDEN RULE

Service and the World

"No kind action ever stops with itself. One kind action leads to another. Good example is followed. A single act of kindness throws out roots in all directions, and the roots spring up and make new trees. The greatest work that kindness does to others is that it makes them kind themselves."

~ Amelia Earhart

In the movie "Evan Almighty", they use a neat little acronym: ARK - Act of Random Kindness. God tells Evan that the way to change the world is by doing one Act of Random Kindness at a time. What an amazing message! Imagine if everyone in the world were to do one act of random kindness at once. That would be like dropping an atomic bomb of kindness on this planet. And I believe if everyone possessed the habit of service, this place would become heaven on earth for all.

(Please take a look and read number VIII and XI of the Code of Ethics. Napoleon Hill knew the benefits of service and the disasters of selfishness. With service the world reaps progressive growth and with selfishness the world reaps most of its troubles.)

Summary of the Benefits of Service

1. Sowing seeds of service means you are sowing constructive seeds such as love, joy, and kindness and these things will surely return to you in a like manner

ONE HABIT AT A TIME

2. When you develop the characteristic of serving others, you will notice that help is more likely to be around when you need it

3. Serving others makes you feel and share the wonderful feelings that they experience from receiving your help

4. Service strengthens your relationship with others and creates powerful relationships that will only increase the chances of success for all parties

5. Service sets an example for others to follow and do the same; the more people that have the habit of service, the closer we will be to experiencing heaven on earth

6. And much more, however; keep in mind that the main focus of service is on benefiting others

HOW TO DEVELOP THE HABIT OF SERVICE

Service and Balance

God has given us the gifts of life and choice. It is now up to us to choose whether or not we wish to give and share as our Creator does. Remember, the habit of service does not mean to neglect your personal desires. It is important to focus on others, but as I have previously recommended, it is also important to focus on personal gains. To focus solely on yourself while neglecting others is one extreme and to focus on others and neglect yourself is the opposite extreme. What is best in life is a balanced focus.

GOLDEN RULE

This book is a great example of a balanced focus of service. It was my personal desire to write a book that I would be proud to claim ownership of. At the same time, it was my intention to create a book that would be of great service to anyone who read and followed it. I believe I have done both. And so can you!

Empowering Relationships

"Some of the biggest challenges in relationships come from the fact that most people enter a relationship in order to get something: they're trying to find someone who's going to make them feel good. In reality, the only way a relationship will last is if you see your relationship as a place that you go to give, and not a place that you go to take."

~ Anthony Robbins

At this point, you have consciously connected to the Source of life. You know that you can always draw from this unlimited Source for anything you desire. Therefore, you should not seek out love, joy or peace from others. All you need to do is draw these things from the Source within and then share them freely with others. In turn, you will notice that others will freely share these things with you.

Service and Receiving

How would you feel: if you kissed someone you love and they did not react; if you went out of your way for a friend and they did not acknowledge your kind actions in anyway; if a colleague at work asked you to take an emergency shift and after doing so, you never hear about this favour you did for them again? As you can see, there is something really important missing. A strong relationship is built on both the giving and receiving of service (love). Remember, receiving well is service too. How does one receive well? There are just as many ways to receive as there are to give. Think about how you would like to see a person react to your service. Here are some common and simple ways to receive service:

- A smile
- A hug
- A kiss
- A heartfelt hand shake
- Giving thanks
- And much more

I believe that if more people learned to recognize and react positively to service, then people would serve more often.

Creating the Habit of Service

"We have committed the Golden Rule to memory; let us now commit it to life."

~Edwin Markham

Beep! The Habit Watch is reminding you to be of service. The first step of service is to focus on something else besides yourself:

- Universal Essence

GOLDEN RULE

- Nature
- A person or people
- A great ideal
- And so on

Once you know what you wish to serve, the second step is to remember the Golden Rule as stated here by Jesus: *"Therefore all things whatsoever ye would that men should do to you, do ye even so to them."* Put yourself in the place of that which you wish to serve and determine what it is that you would like to do. Here are some types of service:

- A positive thought
- A blessing
- A greeting (i.e. "Hello")
- A genuine compliment
- A prayer
- A visualization of a positive outcome
- Giving some positive reinforcement
- And so on

SMILE

"The giving is the hardest part; what does it cost to add a smile?"

~ Jean de la Bruyere

When a smile comes from the heart, the smile itself is a service. As you learned in chapter 3, an authentic smile is welcoming, contagious, and it lights up the world. When you give with a smile, you are communicating that you are joyous in your service. A smile shows that you are giving from your Spirit and not out of an obligation of some sort. So remember, when you serve others, do it with a genuine smile.

A Helpful Perspective

"To keep the Golden Rule we must put ourselves in other people's places, but to do that consists in and depends upon picturing ourselves in their places."

~ Harry Emerson Fosdick

The perspective of "putting yourself in other peoples' places" strongly supports the habit of service. Sometimes we are so focused on our own selves that we forget about the people around us. We are so preoccupied with our own wants and needs that we do not think of the wants and needs of others. If we were to just shift this focus from time to time toward others, we would learn to see their wants and needs. Once we figure out the wants and needs of others, we will find plenty of opportunity for service.

A smile, greeting, and compliment are generic services that everyone usually enjoys receiving. However, sometimes you may also want to personalize a service, so here is how this is done. First of all, you must select the person(s) you wish to serve. Secondly, you must ask "what do they really enjoy?" Finally, go ahead and do the service.

Here is an example. Someone offers you a free pair of tickets for a hockey game. You are not at all interested in hockey. However, instead of declining the offer, you can accept the tickets gratefully and then think of someone to give them to who would be very interested in going to the game. Needless to say, the person(s) receiving these tickets will be ecstatic for your service.

Emotionalize the Habit

"The spirit in which a thing is given determines that in which the debt is acknowledged; it's the intention, not the face-value of the gift, that's weighed."

~ Seneca

When service is done with the intention of goodness, it nourishes the spirit of both the giver and the receiver. In addition, the more love or goodness that is put into a service, the more value it carries. In other words, the value of service is measured by the amount of SPIRIT (or love) we give to others. This is great news because we are all made of spirit and we have an infinite amount to give out. So before you give someone a gift (service), remember to wrap it up with goodness, love and spirit.

Summary of Creating the Habit of Service

- Focus on developing the new habit instead of focusing on breaking the old habit

- Set the Habit Watch to beep once every 15, 30, or 60 minutes

ONE HABIT AT A TIME

- When the Habit Watch goes off, check all previously learned habits and focus on serving something else besides yourself

- Remember the Golden Rule when deciding your service

- Learn to recognize service so that you may receive it greatly

- Put yourself in other peoples' places and do something for them that they would really enjoy

- Ensure to wrap up your service with lots of love, goodness and spirit

- To master the habit practice it for at least 30 days

- You have mastered the habit when you catch yourself practicing it at least 80% of the time

CONCLUSION

Serve and Be Served!

Congratulations! You are NOW ready to use the Habit Watch to develop the habit of service. It is time for you to not only live your purpose but to help others live theirs. It is time for you to give back for all that you have received in your life. And finally, it is time for you to give to others with SPIRIT so that we can all experience heaven on earth!

GOLDEN RULE

Habit 9 – Serve others freely and wrap up your service with love while doing so.

After 30 consecutive days of mastering the habit of service, you will be ready to develop any habit that your heart desires!

Conclusion

YOU ARE ON YOUR WAY!

"No matter how long you live nor how diligent you are, you will never exhaust the supply of new good habits that it is possible to form, nor the supply of old bad habits it is possible to break."

~ Henry Hanzlitt

    Once you have mastered the habits in this book, I promise you that your life will be a lot richer in body, mind, and spirit. However, I do not want you to feel as if the habits in this book are the only habits worth adopting. I could list countless habits that you could develop to improve your life. And you could find all these habits in an endless amount of books written by phenomenal authors from both the past and present. What is exciting is that you now have a practical and easy-to-use method for developing and incorporating any great habit into your life!

    In truth, my vision is that this book will become a fundamental tool for all other self-development books. If this is your first self-development book, I urge you, as I

CONCLUSION

have done before, to continue to read, grow and practice. If you already have some favourite self-development books in your personal library, then you could use the Habit Watch Method to develop the habits in those books as well. As you re-read each book, make a list of the habits you think would benefit you most. Use this same technique for any new self-development books you read there after.

Which Habits Should I Choose To Develop?

"Cultivate only the habits that you are willing should master you."

~ Elbert Hubbard

Falling into a state of unconsciousness is a common habit and it is bound to happen to most people throughout the day. Therefore, I have chosen 9 habits that I believe will be great masters if you do fall into a state of unconsciousness. Would you not want to be mastered by habits such as good posture, accurate thinking and service? In addition, I have chosen the habit of mindfulness which is the exact opposite of unconsciousness. With mindfulness, YOU are the master, thus you cultivate the habits of your choosing. And you should only choose the habits that will lead you to your heart's desires. So remember, the most important thing is to mindfully choose and cultivate the habits that will lead you to your heart's desire.

Note: You can stay up-to-date on the latest habit development news by visiting: **www.habitwatch.ca.**

ONE HABIT AT A TIME

Can I Use The Habit Watch To Rid Conscious Habits?

"A nail is driven out by another nail. Habit is overcome by habit."

~ **Desiderius Erasmus**

The Habit Watch Method can be used for any unconscious habit you wish to develop or rid. But what about conscious habits, can the Habit Watch Method be used to rid those types of habits? The Habit Watch works best for the type of habits that sneak up on us. Its purpose is to get you to a conscious state of mind where you can then make a conscious choice. Therefore, if you are consciously choosing to partake in a certain habit, the Habit Watch Method cannot help you. For instance, if you have the habit of smoking, then you are making a conscious choice to do so.

What can you do then to rid your conscious habits? It is my strong belief that I have presented tremendously powerful habits in this book. By developing these habits, ridding those conscious habits such as smoking will be much easier to accomplish. How do the habits in this book help you rid the conscious habits? The following is a sample chart which explains how each habit may help you to rid the negative habit of smoking:

CONCLUSION

SMOKING HABIT CHART

	Positive Habit From This Book	Traits and Benefits of Habit	Possible Causes of Negative Habit	How Habit Can Help Change Negative Habit
P H Y S I C A L	Good Posture	Confidence	Insecurities	Confidence alleviates insecurities
	High-Quality Breathing	Relaxation	Stress	Relaxation alleviates stress
	Smiling	Joy	Depression	Joy alleviates depression
M E N T A L	Mindfulness	Heightened senses	False sense of feeling good (temporary)	Able to smell, taste, and feel negative effects
	Accurate Thinking	Know and committed to heart's desires	Detached from purpose, ideals, or core values	Smoking is not part of heart's desire (avoided)
	Affirmative Action	Faith	Believe they cannot quit	Have the belief in themselves needed to quit
S P I R I T U A L	Conscious Unity	Spiritual Power	Disconnected to their Spirit	A new source of strength that can be used to quit
	Giving Thanks	Life is a perfect gift perspective	Life is too… (complaint)	Cherish all that you have (body, planet, life, etc.)
	Service	Love for others, planet, etc.	Do not care about others' health	Love for others negates them from smoking

ONE HABIT AT A TIME

As you can see, developing the habits of this book will better prepare you to rid any conscious habit (smoking, over-indulgence of alcoholic beverages, over-eating etc.). Bear in mind, I have only listed one possibility in each box.

Who Can Use The Habit Watch Method And This Book?

"I know of no more encouraging fact than the unquestionable ability of man to elevate his life by conscious endeavor."

~ Henry David Thoreau

I believe that this book and the Habit Watch Method can be used by:

- anyone who has the ability to learn
- anyone who has room for development
- anyone who wants to be richer in body, mind, spirit and life

In other words, EVERYONE! Yes, I envision anyone using this method. It is similar to the alarm clock. Anyone can make use of it and a lot of people do. I believe the Habit Watch will be the 'new' alarm clock. It will be the alarm clock that wakes everyone up from unconsciousness and into a higher state of living. This will lead to a richer and more heavenly life experience for everyone. However, in order for this to happen, I will need you to help spread the word about the Habit Watch and pass on this priceless message of awareness to everyone you know and care about.

CONCLUSION

Also, I envision health and wellness practitioners of all types using this book and the Habit Watch Method on their clients. These are some examples of how the Habit Watch Method can be used to help their clients:

- Holistic Health Practitioners can help their clients develop the many principles and habits of holistic health and living

- Yoga instructors can use this method to help their clients practice awareness, posture and breathing

- CHEK Practitioners can help their clients build the CHEK fundamental principles for a healthier lifestyle

- Chiropractors and Osteopaths can help their clients build good habits for spinal health

- Doctors, Naturopathic/Homeopathic Doctors and Nutritionists can help their clients build a variety of nutritional and lifestyle habits

- Dentists and TMJ Practitioners can help their clients rid the habits of teeth clenching and grinding

And finally, I envision YOU making the most of yourself and living life to the fullest!

Thank you for reading this book and...

ONE HABIT AT A TIME

…LIVE LONG AND PROSPER!

CONCLUSION

Have Your Say:

I would like to hear your feedback on the book and about any experiences you have had building new habits. Please send me your thoughts at **sal_crispo@habitwatch.ca**.

Thank you!

With Love and Respect,

Sal Crispo